Asthma

Answers at your fingertips

FIFTH EDITION

Asthma
Answers at your fingertips

FIFTH EDITION

**Dr Mark L Levy, Monica Fletcher OBE
and Professor Søren Pedersen**

CLASS HEALTH • LONDON

Printing history
First published 1993; reprinted 1993, 1994; Revised edition 1994; reprinted 1996;
Second edition 1997; reprinted 1997; Third edition 2000; Fourth edition 2006;
Fifth edition 2014; Revised reprint 2017

The authors and publisher welcome feedback from the users of this book. Please
contact the publisher.

**Class Health, The Exchange, Express Park, Bristol Road, Bridgwater,
Somerset TA6 4RR
Tel: 44 (0)1278 427800; Fax: 44 (0)1278 421077
Email: post@class.co.uk
www.classhealth.co.uk**

The information presented in this book is accurate and current to the best of the
authors' knowledge. The authors and publisher, however, make no guarantee as
to, and assume no responsibility for, the correctness, sufficiency or completeness
of such information or recommendation. The reader is advised to consult a doctor
regarding all aspects of individual health care.

A CIP catalogue record for this book is available from the British Library.

ISBN: Paperback 978 1 85959 372 1
ISBN: ePub 979 1 85959 373 8

Edited by Gillian Clarke
Cartoons by Jenny Hartree
Line illustrations by David Woodroffe
Typeset by Mach 3 Solutions Ltd, Stroud, Gloucestershire
Printed in the UK by Bell & Bain Ltd, Glasgow

Contents

Introduction

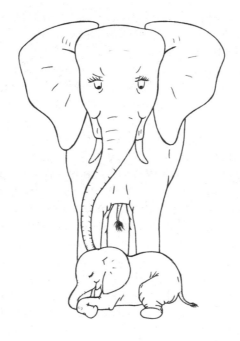

WHAT THIS BOOK IS ABOUT

Asthma is one of the most common long-term conditions, and around 350 million people in the world have it. Health experts working in the field of asthma produce regular updated international guidelines for its management. They agree that people with asthma need information and education about their condition. This should be aimed at individual needs and backed up with written personal asthma action plans (also called PAAPs). There are certain basic principles and skills that need to be understood, however mild the asthma is.

This new version of our 'top 100 questions' updates the previous version of our book, and is available in both paper and electronic forms. It still contains basic information about the condition but also has more detail for anyone with more complex asthma, as well as anyone who has had asthma for many years and wants to ask more 'advanced' questions.

We have, however, changed the layout of the chapters to make it easier for you to learn about your own asthma in addition to making it available in electronic form.

As in previous editions, this 5th edition provides clear answers to real questions from our patients. These answers will be helpful for anyone interested in asthma, particularly people with asthma and their families and friends wanting to understand more about the condition.

To live life to the full, it is essential that you understand how to recognise worsening asthma and prevent asthma attacks. We believe that it is vital for you to be involved in your own care (that is, in 'self-care' or 'self-management'), as you are the person who lives with asthma day in and day out. In this book we provide you with information and practical tips that will enable you to manage your asthma and reduce the problems it can cause you. It is to be used in addition to medical advice from your own doctor or asthma nurse.

In the first chapters, we help you to understand how variable asthma is – how it changes from time to time, and how it affects people. We also explain the things that make asthma worse, so you can try to avoid them. We believe it is important to have a basic understanding of respiratory signs and symptoms and how asthma is diagnosed – this is covered in Chapter 3. It is vital to recognise when you need to worry about asthma, because these same signs and symptoms also occur when asthma goes out of control. So you will know when to take extra asthma medicines or to call for emergency help.

In the sections covering asthma medicines, we have tried to be consistent in the names we have used. There are many brand names for anti-asthma medicines, as well as the true (or generic) names, and we realise that these can be confusing. Where a particular name has been included in the question we continue to use that name (although we might give the generic name, too). You will find more detail about the different medicines and inhaler devices used for asthma in Chapter 4, 'Treatments for asthma'.

Throughout the book you will find references to peak flow meters and peak expiratory flow (PEF) readings. The peak flow meter is a small and simple piece of equipment that measures how hard you can blow (see Figure 5.1 in Chapter 5). When your *airways* are narrowed, such as during an asthma attack, the reading you get on the meter scale will be reduced. When you are well, the reading will be higher. We believe that monitoring the peak expiratory flow, combined with recognising the presence of asthma symptoms, is the best way to keep a check on your asthma (rather like using a machine to measure your blood pressure).

This does not mean that we believe everyone with asthma should be using peak flow meters all the time. But when problems arise, they do give the best assessment of how severe the asthma is. There is a section in Chapter 5, 'Beating asthma', on the use of peak flow meters.

Unfortunately, there is no cure for asthma at the present time. Nevertheless, with a good understanding of your asthma, it is possible to keep your symptoms under excellent control. The information in this book will help you to learn to recognise the danger signs and to treat episodes when it might be getting out of control.

Occupational asthma may either resolve completely or improve a lot once an affected person is no longer exposed to the cause. This depends on how long they were exposed and how severe their symptoms were before being removed from the cause.

Many people are troubled unnecessarily by their asthma because they are not receiving the right treatment, or because they do not realise the benefits of current asthma treatments. Sections in Chapters 5, 6 and 8 provide information on self-management and what to do in asthma emergencies.

Inevitably, some of the terms we use are medical or technical. We have tried to explain these terms wherever they occur, and to steer clear of medical jargon. We have also included a glossary of some of the more important (and perhaps confusing) medical terms that tend to come up time and time again. When these terms are first mentioned in the book, we have italicised them; for example, *bronchial hyperreactivity*.

HOW TO BEAT YOUR ASTHMA

The major challenge is to find ways of living with asthma without the illness interfering too much with daily life. For some people, having asthma is a problem, and people solve problems in different ways. In this book, we support a problem-solving approach, initially by making sure that you have the information you need.

Problem solving has several stages.

- It begins with identifying or clarifying a particular problem (e.g. your asthma is making you breathless when you run), and then trying to imagine where you want to be in the future (e.g. to be able to run without getting breathless).

- The next stage is to figure out how you are going to get from where you are to where you want to be. Gathering information allows you to find out as much as you can about the cause of the problem and how to fix it.

- Next you see how this information applies to you (e.g. you might want to prove that your asthma is indeed the cause of your breathlessness, perhaps by using a peak flow meter).

- Finally you find ways of using this information to solve the problem (e.g. agreeing a personal asthma action plan with your doctor or asthma nurse).

Each chapter starts with a number of learning points so that you can focus your thoughts on these while reading the chapter. We suggest that, as you read through the book, you think about questions that are important for you, and write them down. You may wish to ask your doctor or asthma nurse these questions when you next go to see them. We also end each chapter with a number of suggested questions. In this way, we hope to give you a structured approach to finding out about asthma and using what you learn to help you live a life unrestricted by it.

HOW TO USE THIS BOOK

Because people have differing needs for information about asthma, this book has been designed so that you do not have to read it from cover to cover. The questions and their answers are arranged into chapters and sections; you may want to dip into sections, or look for the answer to a particular question by using the contents list.

If you have just been diagnosed as having asthma, we suggest that you concentrate on the following sections first:

- 'What is asthma?' in Chapter 1

- 'Symptoms' and 'Triggers' in Chapter 2

- 'Medicines' in Chapter 4

- 'Emergencies' in Chapter 8.

If you are experienced in managing your asthma, you may wish to concentrate more on the peak expiratory flow rate sections in Chapters 3 and 5.

If your child has asthma, we hope that Chapter 7 will deal with many of your concerns.

Inevitably there will be some repetition in the book, and some information will seem to be duplicated in different sections. There is some cross-referencing of answers, but we have tried to keep this to a minimum. We prefer to answer each question in full, rather than direct you to a number of different sections each time, but for reasons of space this is not always possible.

This book has been written from *real* questions that we have been asked by hundreds of *real* people with *real* asthma! Not everyone will agree that the questions we have chosen are the important ones, and certainly not everyone will agree with the answers we have provided. Each edition of this book has been improved by feedback from the people who know most about problems relating to asthma – you! We really hope that you will enjoy this book and find it helpful in controlling your asthma.

If you have any comments about the contents of this book, we will be delighted to receive them. Please write to us, c/o Class Publishing, The Exchange, Express Park, Bristol Road, Bridgwater, Somerset TA6 4RR, UK.

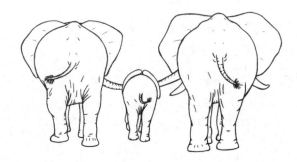

1 | What is asthma and how does it affect people?

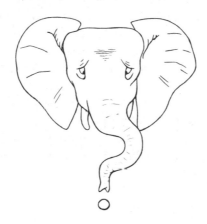

In this chapter you will learn:

- what asthma is

- what happens to your airways when you have asthma

- why people with asthma sometimes die

- the 'hygiene hypothesis'

- the likelihood of inheriting asthma.

Asthma varies in severity in both adults and children. It can be mild, with only an occasional need for treatment, or moderate in that regular treatment is needed for longer periods of time. There is also a smaller number of people who have severe asthma that requires repeated hospital admissions and causes a restricted lifestyle.

Fortunately, many people are able to lead a full life, either free from symptoms or with minimal symptoms. Nevertheless, few health conditions have a greater impact than asthma.

It is estimated that over 350 million people worldwide have asthma, which creates a heavy economic burden in all countries. These costs are related to health care, social security payments in the form of invalidity payments, and lost productivity as a result of sickness and absence from work. About 250,000 deaths in the world are caused by asthma every year, and many of these are preventable

When you are first told that you have asthma, many thoughts will flash through your mind. If you have a close friend or relative with asthma, you will wonder whether your own condition will be like theirs. No two people have the same pattern of symptoms, and even for the same person, symptoms can vary in severity at different times.

The important points to learn about your own asthma are:

- how it affects you

- what makes it worse, and

- how your treatment can help.

Do not be too influenced by what happens to other people – we are all different!

ASTHMA EXPLAINED

What is asthma?

We have two *lungs*, which are like a pair of large bellows (see Figure 1.1). They are situated in our chest and are essential for bringing oxygen from the air into our bloodstream (breathing in) and removing carbon dioxide (breathing out).

The air passages, also called *airways* or *bronchi*, are tubes through which we breathe air in and out of our lungs. Asthma is a condition that causes inflammation (swelling and the production of mucus) and tightening and narrowing of the air passages, which makes

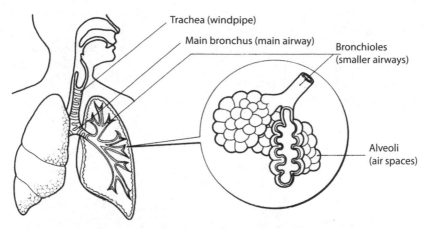

Figure 1.1 This is what the lungs look like inside. Air breathed in goes from the windpipe (*trachea*) into the two main airways (*bronchi*; singular = bronchus). From there it goes through the small tubes (*bronchioles*) to the lung's air spaces (*alveoli*) and then is absorbed into the bloodstream.
© Education for Health; adapted with permission from Education for Health, Warwick (www.educationforhealth.org)

breathing difficult. This occasional or intermittent tightening is characteristic of asthma. Most people are fit and well in between attacks or episodes, and can breathe normally.

It might be easier to appreciate the structure of the lungs if they are likened to an upside-down tree. Here, the tree trunk is similar to the main windpipe (*trachea*); the larger branches are the main airways (main *bronchi*). The smaller branches resemble the smaller airways (still called *bronchi*) and the twigs represent the very small airways (*bronchioles*). The leaves represent the air sacs (*alveoli*).

Air is breathed in through the nose and mouth and into the main windpipe (trachea). Air then travels though the larger branches (the main bronchi) and to smaller branches (the bronchi) and then to even smaller airways (bronchioles). At the end of the air passages the air reaches the air sacs (alveoli). It is in the air sacs that oxygen passes from the air into the bloodstream, and the waste product – carbon dioxide – is passed in the opposite direction, out of the blood into the air sacs. This is known as gas exchange or respiration.

If you have asthma, it will affect your bronchi. They become narrow, which makes it more difficult for air to move to and from the air sacs (see Figure 1.2). Asthma is sometimes referred to as 'bronchial asthma'.

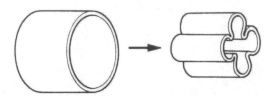

a Tightening of airways from muscle spasm with reduced space

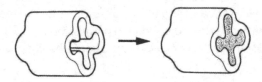

b Swelling of walls, with production of thick mucus

Figure 1.2 In asthma, the (normal) airways narrow owing to spasm (tightening) of the muscles around them and swelling of their lining and sticky mucus inside them.

© Education for Health; adapted with permission from Education for Health, Warwick (www.educationforhealth.org)

TYPES OF ASTHMA

Is my asthma caused by an allergy?

*A*sthma and *allergy* are not the same thing but they do often go together. If you have an allergy, your body has an over-sensitive response to something (or things) that many people have no reaction to.

If you are allergic to something that you breathe in, it can cause symptoms of *wheezing*, itchy mouth and lips or a runny nose. Allergies can also make your eyes run and itch. The substances that trigger an *allergic reaction* are known as *allergens*. An allergic reaction does not happen the first time you come into contact with a particular allergen. It usually develops over a period of time after subsequent or repeat exposure to the allergen.

Grass pollen, *house dust mite*, pet hair, foods, perfumes and colourings are just some of the everyday things that can cause an allergic reaction in some people.

Asthma is often triggered by an allergic reaction. For example, if you are allergic to cats, just handling, stroking or even being in the same room as one can produce asthma symptoms either immediately or a few hours later.

Sometimes it is easy to identify the allergen that triggers asthma symptoms; at other times it is very difficult. Once the allergen has been identified, avoiding or reducing the amount of contact with that asthma trigger is sensible but it is not always easy to do so.

My doctor talks about different types of asthma. What does this mean?

*T*here are different types of asthma depending on what has triggered the condition, and may or may not be a result of an allergic response. Asthma can be triggered by:

- allergy
- exercise

- infection
- hormone changes
- an irritant
- environmental factors.

Asthma varies greatly in severity. When it is mild and infrequent, it is referred to as 'episodic' or 'occasional'. At other times asthma may be persistent (*chronic*) or severe. Mild or episodic asthma is usually triggered by the common cold.

Asthma commonly starts in childhood, though it may occur at any stage in life. When asthma starts in adulthood, it is referred to as *late-onset asthma*. In addition, people may develop asthma symptoms due to specific triggers such as the following.

- **Exercise or excessive exertion** Exercise is a common asthma trigger, and some people only ever have asthma symptoms after some sort of exercise. If someone exercises infrequently, reliever inhaler medicine immediately beforehand is likely to be the only treatment required. If someone does a lot of exercise, though, asthma symptoms will be more frequent, and likely to be more of a nuisance. In this situation, regular use of a *preventer* (sometimes called a 'controller') and a *reliever* asthma inhaler when needed will control asthma symptoms better than just a reliever (the medical term is 'bronchodilator').

- **Occupation** *Occupational asthma* is so called because it is caused or made worse by the person's work environment. (If asthma has been made worse by exposure to substances at work, it is known as *work-aggravated asthma*.) If your asthma gets better when you are not at work, we suggest you tell your doctor, because you may need to see a specialist. Some additional tests may be needed to identify the trigger.

- **In the hay fever (pollen) season** Pollen asthma, as the name suggests, happens in the pollen or *hay fever* season. This will occur at different times of the year depending on where you live. Hay fever belongs to the group of conditions called *allergic rhinitis*, but in this case it would be triggered specifically by the pollen.

Asthma triggered by pollen will be seasonal. The pollen season lasts from early spring right through to the end of the summer but there are three phases, which may overlap, depending on where you live:

- early or late spring as a result of tree pollens

- in summer as a result of grass pollens

- in the summer through autumn as a result of mould spores.

Although pollen is a common asthma trigger, few people are unlucky enough to be troubled through all three phases of the pollen season.

If asthma symptoms do not happen at any other time of the year, asthma treatment can be started a few weeks before the known pollen trigger and continued for as long as it is around.

I have no relatives with asthma, and now at the age of 42 years I have developed it. Why me?

Asthma is very common, developing in about 1 in 20 (5%) of adults. It may develop at any age and sometimes there is no inherited factor. Just as asthma can be triggered by a *virus* infection (such as a cold) in young children, it can also be triggered by a respiratory infection later in life. It is possible that this is what has happened to you, but it is also possible that your asthma is due to 'occupational exposure'. If you are working in one of the occupations associated with asthma, you should ask your doctor or nurse to check for this (see the question 'What is occupational asthma?' in Chapter 6).

If you had asthma as a child, it is possible that it has returned. Asthma in childhood is sometimes not diagnosed, especially if the respiratory symptoms are mild; they are often referred to as 'bronchitis' or 'chestiness'. These respiratory symptoms tend to improve and settle down later in childhood but for some reason recur later on in adult life; this might have happened with you.

Throughout this book we emphasise that the severity of asthma varies enormously. Many people feel very worried and anxious when they are told that they have asthma; others feel disbelief or are angry. However, once they know more about their asthma and the fact that it can be treated successfully, most find that these feelings go away and they come to terms with their condition.

Having asthma can still carry an unnecessary stigma and some people feel ashamed and don't want anyone to know about it. Fortunately, modern asthma treatments help you to be free from symptoms at all times and able to lead a full life with no restrictions on what you can do. So you shouldn't feel stigmatised or different. It is so common that most people know someone with the condition.

ABOUT ASTHMA

Is asthma catching? Can I give it to my children?

You cannot 'catch' asthma because it is not an infectious disease. However, some people think it is because:

- you *can* catch a cold, which may make asthma worse

- asthma and allergic conditions often run in families (see the section on inheritance, page 17), and some people believe that asthma is an infectious disease

- asthma is more common now and people believe (wrongly) that the disease is 'spreading' like an infectious disease.

One of the strongest explanations for the recent rise in allergic diseases – and asthma is one of these – is the so-called 'hygiene hypothesis'. This theory, which has been around for some time, states that people exposed to lots of different infective organisms are protected from developing allergic diseases. For example, people raised in a farming environment are exposed to a variety of organisms and suffer less from allergic disease. When we live in much cleaner environments, we don't build up resistance to such conditions.

Can asthma be cured?

No, asthma cannot be cured but it can be controlled by effective treatment. The symptoms may be alleviated totally with effective treatment, and may sometimes disappear even without treatment.

Asthma is therefore called a variable condition. There are times when people feel that they must be cured because they are completely without symptoms. While this symptomless state (called *remission*) can go on for a long time, once you have had asthma you will always have the potential to have it again, even years later.

It is probably better to think of asthma going into remission rather than being cured.

I read in the local paper that someone had died as a result of an asthma attack. Why does this happen?

Because asthma is so common, it is easy to think 'it's only asthma', but it is important to know that asthma can have very serious consequences. While deaths from asthma are not very common, many of these sad events are associated with potentially preventable factors and might therefore have been avoided. Many deaths happen in people with uncontrolled asthma, and therefore it is vital to have your asthma checked regularly, especially if you are needing to use more that one reliever inhaler a month. It is also vital to take your preventer inhaler regularly as directed by your doctor or nurse.

In order to prevent asthma attacks and possible death:

- Have an agreed personal asthma action plan (ask your doctor or nurse for one)

- Take your asthma seriously

- Make sure you collect regular preventer inhaler prescriptions

- Take your medication regularly

- Attend asthma check-ups

- Find out how to tell if your asthma is out of control

- Call for medical help urgently if your asthma is out of control

A small number of people have very severe and unstable asthma despite taking their asthma medicines. This is called *brittle asthma* or chronic severe asthma. Occasionally, some deaths do occur in this group because of the seriousness of their asthma.

Do children die from asthma?

Children can die from asthma but thankfully this is very rare. However, when a child's death could have been prevented it is tragic.

Two groups of children are at particular risk. In one group are those who have both asthma and food allergy (e.g. peanut allergy), especially if they are prone to sudden severe allergic reactions, known as *anaphylaxis*. These children should be under the care of a specialist with expertise in asthma and allergy. The other group at risk are teenagers as they start to exert their authority in life. They may, as a result, stop taking their medications regularly and don't see asthma as being an important part of their lives.

Very rarely, children do die as a result of their first asthma attack. They may have had very minor asthma symptoms in the past, which might have been ignored or not thought of as serious. Fortunately, such deaths are extremely rare. Nevertheless, for many parents, this often leaves them with the unanswered question: 'Could I have done something to prevent my child's death?'

In childhood, the parents' knowledge, beliefs and commitment to the treatment are just as important as the child's own reaction to asthma.

INHERITANCE

Why do I have asthma?

There is not always a clear answer to this reasonable question! People may wonder why they have asthma, but others almost expect it because it runs so strongly in their families. We know that some of our characteristics (such as the colour of our eyes) and some rare diseases (such as haemophilia) can be caused by inheriting single *genes* but it is likely that a number of different genes play a role in the 'asthma tendency'. Research involving twins and families, and the discovery of the ADAM33 gene, has found a genetic link with asthma. In other words, asthma may run in your family.

Some people with an inherited tendency to develop asthma may go through their entire lives and not develop it, despite encountering trigger factors many times. This is just one more mystery showing how much we still don't understand about the cause of asthma. They may, however, have other allergic (*atopic*) manifestations such as *eczema* or hay fever, but no respiratory symptoms.

Viral infections of the respiratory system (e.g. the common cold) usually set off changes in the linings of the airways, leading to asthma symptoms; for other people, allergies are the trigger. Adults in certain occupations may also develop asthma as a result of substances they come into contact with at work.

As asthma runs in families, is there anything I can do to prevent my children from getting it?

One factor we do know about is exposure to second-hand tobacco smoke. Children of parents who smoke are more likely to develop asthma, and very likely to suffer from exposure to the smoke – so there is a clear message there!

There is some evidence to suggest that children who are exposed to allergy-causing substances in the first few months of life are more likely to develop asthma later in childhood, particularly if there is a history of allergy in the family as well.

There is confusing information about breastfeeding and whether it protects your baby against asthma or other atopic (allergic) conditions such as eczema. From the different scientific information, it seems that breastfeeding may be helpful in preventing the development of allergic diseases. In any case, breastfed children tend to have fewer viral infections, and suffer less from eczema than those who are not breastfed; so it is beneficial.

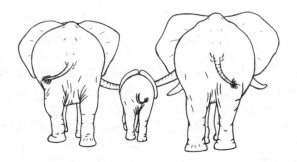

2 | Symptoms and triggers of asthma

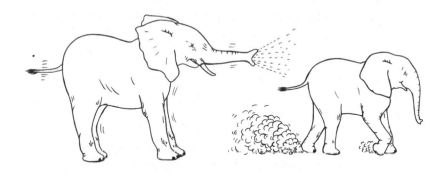

In this chapter you will learn about:

- asthma symptoms
- how asthma symptoms make your asthma worse
- asthma triggers
- how asthma triggers make your asthma worse.

SYMPTOMS

What are the symptoms of asthma?

The main symptoms of asthma are:

- **Coughing** When the airways are irritated and sensitive (*twitchy*), this can make you cough. The coughing is often worse at night. Common colds often cause coughing for 2–4 weeks. Frequent slight coughing is seen in most people with asthma.

- **Wheezing** When the airways in the lungs become tight, they narrow in size. This makes it more difficult to breathe out normally and air has to be forced out. If air is forced out of the lungs through narrowed airways, it causes a high-pitched squeaky or whistling noise known as *wheezing*. The wheezing can be heard because the space in the airways (the 'calibre') has been reduced by 40% or more (nearly half the width).

- **Chest tightness and heavy breathing** When the airways become narrow, it can give you the feeling that there is something tight around your chest, and this makes breathing uncomfortable. It can be quite painful too and, because of this, you may think something is wrong with your heart, but asthma does not affect the heart in this way.

- **Shortness of breath** When the airways are tight, breathing is harder than normal and results in shortness of breath, especially during work or exercise.

Can I get rid of my asthma symptoms?

It is not possible to get rid of your asthma but it is certainly possible to get rid of your symptoms.

Symptoms are a reflection of poor asthma control. People with good asthma control have no or few symptoms, so this is what you and your doctor or asthma nurse should aim for. With correct treatment, the vast majority of patients can achieve good asthma control.

Asthma control is normally graded from good to poor. There are several ways to help you to assess whether your asthma is controlled. The easiest is to ask yourself four questions:

1. Am I able to do as much physical activity as other people my age?

2. Am I getting asthma symptoms, such as cough, wheeze or shortness of breath, during the day?

3. Am I getting asthma symptoms, such as cough, wheeze or shortness of breath, during the night?

4. Am I using my reliever inhaler (usually coloured blue) more than twice a week?

If you answer Yes to any of these questions, your asthma is out of control. If you check your lung function – for example, with a peak flow meter – you may get additional information on your asthma control. If the reading is 20% lower than usual, your asthma is definitely out of control.

You may also do a formal asthma control test by going online to www.asthma.com/additional-resources/asthma-control-test.html or you could direct your doctor or nurse to the control test on the GINA Report website at www.ginasthma.org

If your asthma is poorly controlled, you should see your doctor and start treatment or, if you are already having treatment, have your asthma medicines adjusted. If you have a personal asthma action plan you should start using it as directed by your doctor. Symptoms are not 'normal'. Having symptoms only three times a week does not mean that your asthma is controlled most of the time (the four days with no symptoms). This is because many people with asthma adjust their life to prevent symptoms, even though they may not be fully aware they are doing this. Their symptom-free days are achieved by placing restrictions in their lifestyle (no sports, staying home in bad weather, not going where people smoke, etc.). Think carefully about what you avoid in your daily life to prevent asthma symptoms!

Asthma symptoms and lung function vary over time. This variability is typical for asthma. The greater the variability, the more uncontrolled is the asthma. Controlled asthma is characterised by having no or little variability – like being healthy with no symptoms or restrictions most of the time.

Below is a summary of various reasons why poorly controlled asthma should be avoided:

Poor daily asthma control is associated with:

- a high risk of having asthma attacks and the need to use *oral steroids* (cortisone or prednisolone)

- an increased risk of having to be hospitalised because of asthma

- reduced quality of life

- restrictions in lifestyle (not doing sports, losing time at work and missing school days)

- increased health-care costs

- worsening lung function over time

- less daily physical activity

- increased risk of obesity

- poorer fitness

- higher risk of anxiety and depression.

TRIGGERS

Do asthma triggers cause asthma?

Generally speaking, asthma triggers do not *cause* asthma – they bring on asthma symptoms or attacks – particularly in people with uncontrolled asthma. An exception is occupational triggers, which may actually cause asthma in some people. (See the question 'What is occupational asthma?' in Chapter 6.)

My son is 6 years old and has asthma. Why does a cold always go to his chest?

Most people with asthma will be familiar with the cold that 'goes to the chest'. Colds are more common in the autumn and winter, and they are caused by virus infections that affect the upper respiratory airway system – the nose and throat. This stays as a 'head cold' for many people, but others, especially those with asthma, find that they quite rapidly develop chesty symptoms.

In children, colds are the most common trigger for making asthma worse. Colds cannot be avoided, but the chest symptoms will be markedly reduced if you ensure that your son's asthma is controlled – the longer the asthma is controlled, the fewer the chest symptoms. Sometimes the only chest symptom will be an increase in cough for a couple of weeks.

I developed asthma when I was 45 years old. No one in my family has ever had asthma before, so what do you think is the likely cause?

S ome people develop asthma later in life, just as you have done, and normally we do not know why. Sometimes a heavy cold 'goes to your chest' and can be the initial trigger of the asthma symptoms.

Another cause of *late-onset asthma* is occupational asthma. There are a number of industries where there is increased risk of developing occupational asthma. This may begin with rhinitis (runny, itchy nose with sneezing), which starts after beginning a new job. There is more about occupational asthma in Chapters 5 and 6.

If you are working in an industry known to be associated with risks of developing occupational asthma, you should ask your doctor or asthma nurse for further tests.

What is passive smoking, and why is it bad for you?

P *assive smoking* is breathing in air polluted by tobacco smoke from other people. If you have asthma, passive smoking is likely to make it worse because the tiny smoke particles in the air irritate the lungs and cause increased asthma symptoms.

Passive smoking is bad because it can irritate your airways even if you do not have asthma. Many pubs, clubs and restaurants are aware of the risks of passive smoking. That is why smoking in these places has been banned in many countries, either voluntarily or by law.

When I tried to buy some aspirin, the chemist asked me if I had asthma. Why?

We know that certain medicines can make asthma worse. The most important group of these medicines is called the non-steroidal *anti-inflammatory drugs* (or *NSAIDs*); aspirin is one of these. Similar medicines include: ibuprofen (Nurofen, Junifen), indometacin and diclofenac (Voltarol). Not everybody is aspirin-sensitive but the pharmacist is quite right to be cautious. People with nasal *polyps* (swellings in the nose) are more likely to react to these medicines and therefore they should avoid taking them. Aspirin and the other NSAIDs can cause serious, sometimes life-threatening, asthma attacks, mainly in adults.

As you are probably aware, aspirin and many of the other NSAIDs are available without prescription and can be purchased in the supermarket or local pharmacy. These medicines are taken by lots of people for headaches, period pains, joint pains and other aches and pains. Aspirin is also taken every day (in a low dose) by people at risk of stroke or heart attack.

Allergic reactions to NSAIDs are rare in children.

I have asthma. If I can't take aspirin, is it OK to take paracetamol (acetaminophen)?

Yes it is, but there have been some reports that asthma can be made worse if you take paracetamol. One of the difficulties here is that paracetamol is usually used when a child has a fever, and this generally means the child has an infection which can itself make the asthma worse. So it's difficult to know what is causing the worsening asthma – is it the infection or the paracetamol? In time, when the results of research on this subject are known, it may become clear.

From the evidence doctors have, the advice is that paracetamol is safe to take, as long as you keep within the recommended doses. However, if you feel that your asthma is made worse by paracetamol, you should not take it. Do talk to your local pharmacist or your asthma nurse or doctor about alternative pain relief.

Why do some things such as cat hairs set off my asthma symptoms, but other pet hairs (e.g. dog hairs) do not?

We do not know the complete answer here. There is so much variation between individuals that it is impossible to cover all the factors involved. Not everyone is allergic to the same substances and just what triggers your asthma will depend on your particular allergy.

Domestic pets often live close to us, and their hair or dander or feathers – even skin, saliva or urine – can trigger asthma symptoms.

Cats are the most common trigger of animal allergy, particularly in children. Many people are allergic only to kittens, or to certain breeds, particularly Siamese and Burmese. Dogs, horses, hamsters and guinea-pigs can also cause allergic asthma.

Although hair and shed skin cells are often responsible for the allergy, surprisingly it has been shown that the allergen is in the cat's saliva. When the animal washes itself, the allergen sticks to hairs, allowing easier contact with the person with asthma.

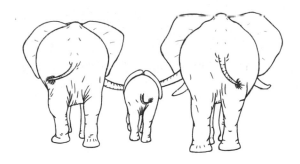

3 | How is asthma diagnosed?

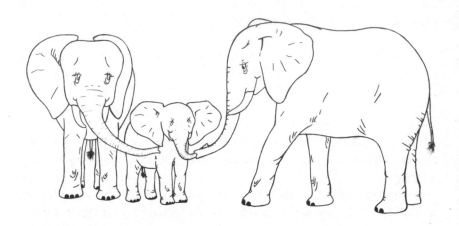

In this chapter you will learn:

- how asthma is diagnosed
- the symptoms of asthma
- how it affects people
- how to look after yourself if you have asthma
- how to know when asthma is getting worse
- how to prevent asthma attacks
- other respiratory (breathing) conditions that may be confused with asthma.

When people go to see a health professional because of breathing problems, or coughing or wheezing, it suggests that there is a respiratory (lung) cause.

Breathing problems are frequently called respiratory symptoms and are mainly:

- coughing

- wheezing (which is a whistling or squeaking sound coming from the chest)

- shortness of breath.

These symptoms are often due to infections caused by the 'common cold'. Colds are the result of viral infections and in most people they get better in 1–2 weeks without any drug treatment.

The same symptoms, however, also occur in asthma, and they may differ from person to person. Some people may get cough or wheeze or shortness of breath, or a combination of these.

The big question is whether you are suffering from repeated chest infections or if the infections are causing asthma to flare up. Things that cause asthma to flare up are called asthma *triggers*, and colds and other infections are known to do this.

If you have an infection you may:

- feel ill quite quickly

- have a raised temperature, or fever

- have a runny nose

- sometimes cough up phlegm, which is thick and sticky and a greenish colour.

Chest infections do not often recur in the same person. So anyone needing to see a doctor more than two or three times a year for repeated respiratory symptoms is likely to have asthma, until proved otherwise.

Asthma symptoms can be triggered by:

- a common cold or other infection

- pollen in the air such as in the *hay fever* season
- dust
- some foods (nuts, kiwi fruit)
- smoky atmospheres
- perfumes or strong smells.

Making the diagnosis of asthma can sometimes be difficult, but the main clue is that asthma symptoms come and go. So a person with asthma may be well and fit at one moment, and severely short of breath at another.

Some people have an inherited chance of developing asthma. The clue to this is whether anyone in the family has asthma. A *family history* of asthma, or other allergic conditions such as hay fever (allergic rhinitis), *eczema*, allergy to food or medicines (such as penicillin or other antibiotics), means that there is a greater risk of someone developing any of these conditions.

A factor that increases the chance of a child getting asthma is if one or both parents smoke.

DIAGNOSIS OF ASTHMA – TESTS AND INVESTIGATIONS

What sorts of tests are done to see if asthma is the problem?

Once asthma is suspected by your doctor or nurse, the diagnosis needs to be confirmed. This is so that:

- the correct treatment can be prescribed
- an action plan for managing your asthma can be agreed between you and your doctor or nurse.

Knowing how to prevent an asthma attack and understanding what triggers your asthma can also be discussed once the diagnosis has been made.

There are three ways of confirming the diagnosis of asthma:

- from the clues in the person's *medical history* – their symptoms and when they occur

- by doing tests that identify whether the airways are becoming narrow (obstructed) during periods of respiratory symptoms (the tests, called Lung Function Tests, are either *peak expiratory flow* tests, using a peak flow meter, or *spirometry* tests using a spirometer)

- by prescribing an anti-asthma medicine and seeing if the symptoms improve.

The diagnosis of asthma is more likely if you also suffer from allergy, eczema or hay fever, or if there are people in the family who also have these conditions.

How do doctors diagnose asthma?

There is more than one way of diagnosing asthma. The medical history on its own is often enough for the diagnosis to be suspected. This should then be confirmed by the doctor or nurse undertaking an assessment of the person's lung function. There are many factors in the past medical history to suggest asthma as the cause of someone's problem.

Asthma is a *chronic* (long-lasting) condition, in which people may be free from symptoms for periods of time and very ill at others. They will usually have a pattern of symptoms that come and go.

Diagnosing asthma can be done in older children and adults by the use of peak flow meter readings or more detailed blowing tests called *spirometry* (described below).

In some cases, as in very young children, when spirometry or peak flow measurements are not possible, the most suitable way of making the diagnosis, together with a detailed medical history, is to see if anti-asthma treatment clears the symptoms. Sometimes this may need to be taken for a number of weeks before it starts to work. This is called a 'trial of therapy' or 'trial of treatment'.

What does my doctor mean when he talks about 'peak expiratory flow' and 'spirometry'?

Asthma is a condition that causes narrowing of the airways, due to:

- spasm (tightening) of the muscle surrounding the airways

- swelling of the airway walls

- increased mucus inside the airways.

'Lung function tests' (e.g. Peak Flow and spirometry) – which test how strongly you can blow air out of your lungs – are used to diagnose asthma and to see if the airways are narrowed. They are:

- the *peak expiratory flow* test (also known as the peak flow or PEF)

- *spirometry*.

Peak flow meters are inexpensive and are usually available on prescription; they are very useful for diagnosing and checking on asthma control. Use of spirometers requires quite a lot of training for doctors and nurses and if used correctly can provide very reliable information.

Both peak expiratory flow and spirometry are used to measure how 'tight' (or narrow) the airways are and to see if the tightness improves after treatment. The tighter (or narrower) the airways are, the lower the peak flow or spirometry readings. These tests are also used to get 'blowing' measurements, or readings, during episodes when people have symptoms and also at other times when there aren't any.

A peak flow diary chart is used to record these readings. In this way, the readings can be compared to see if they change from time to time. In someone who does not have asthma, the readings stay almost the same. In someone with asthma, the PEF readings change (vary) by more than 20% from morning to evening or from day to day.

My doctor has told me to keep a peak flow diary chart.
Why is this?

P eak flow diary charts can be used both to diagnose asthma and to see if someone who already has asthma has it well controlled or not. There are three main patterns of peak flow charts that suggest asthma (or for checking asthma control): they are shown in Figures 3.1, 3.2, 3.3 and 3.4.

The *peak expiratory flow* measures how air flows through the airways. If the airways are narrowed or tightened, as in episodes of asthma, the readings are lower. The measurement of air flow tested using a peak flow meter or a spirometer is given in litres of flow in a minute, written as litres/minute or l/min.

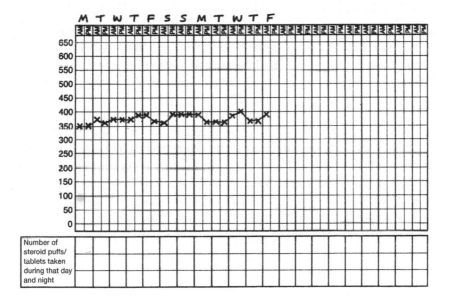

Figure 3.1 A peak flow diary chart showing readings that do not change from day to day. This type of chart is seen either in people who have well-controlled asthma at this time or in those who do not have asthma.

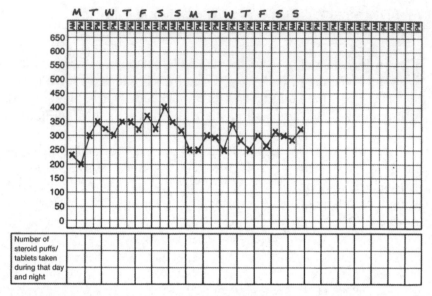

Figure 3.2 A peak flow diary chart showing changing readings (variation) from day to day. In someone with respiratory symptoms, a chart like this would help to confirm the diagnosis of asthma. In someone with asthma, this chart indicates poor control and that more treatment may be needed.

Peak flow readings can vary between good times and bad times. If these vary by more than 20% the diagnosis of asthma is usually confirmed. The 'blowing' test can take place during the consultation with your doctor or nurse but you may be asked to keep a 'peak flow diary' at home.

The important changes that will help doctors and asthma nurses to diagnose asthma from the peak flow diary results are:

- a variation between readings of more than 20% (see Figure 3.2)

- an increased difference between the morning and evening readings (see Figure 3.2)

- an early *morning dip* in the readings (see Figure 3.3).

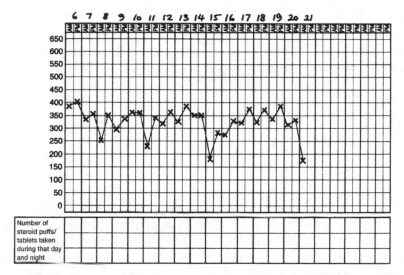

Figure 3.3 A peak flow chart showing early morning 'dipping' in the readings. In someone with symptoms of asthma, a chart like this would help to confirm the diagnosis of asthma. In someone with asthma, this chart indicates poor control and more treatment may be needed. The calculation here is 150/350 × 100 = 42%, so this person has variable obstruction of air flow and therefore probably has asthma.

How are the changes (variation) in peak flow readings worked out?

The changes in peak flow readings can be worked out by the following simple mathematical equation:

$$\frac{\text{Highest PEF reading} - \text{lowest PEF reading}}{\text{Highest PEF reading}} \times 100 = \text{\% change in PEF}$$

The peak flow variability is calculated by using the highest and lowest readings measured in a person during the last few weeks. This can also be done by taking the lowest and highest readings before and after exercise or before and after asthma medication.

For example, if a person's highest peak flow over the previous week was 400 *litres per minute* (l/min), and the lowest was 300 l/min, the calculation of variability would be 25%, as shown below:

$$\frac{\text{Highest PEF reading (400)} - \text{lowest PEF reading (300)}}{\text{Highest PEF reading (400)}} \times 100 = 25\% \text{ change in PEF}$$

How do I tell when my asthma is out of control?

Peak flow charts can help people with diagnosed asthma tell if their asthma is poorly controlled. The peak flow chart in Figure 3.4 shows readings that are dropping from day to day. This person has poorly controlled, deteriorating asthma, and urgent medical help is needed.

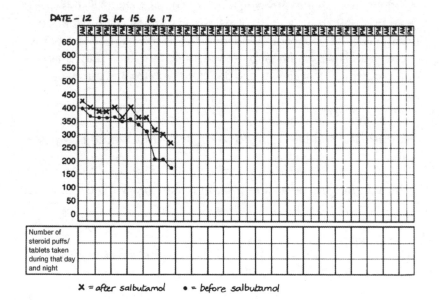

Figure 3.4 Peak flow chart showing readings that are dropping from day to day. This person has poorly controlled, deteriorating asthma.

Do I have to record my peak flow readings on a chart or can I just write them down?

You can write your readings down as in Figure 3.5, which shows how readings can be recorded without using graphs. Here they change from day to day, from 200 to 350 l/min. The calculation is $150/350 \times 100 = 42\%$, showing that this person has variable obstruction of airflow and therefore probably has asthma.

Day	Morning readings (best of 3)	Evening readings (best of 3)
Monday 25th	230	200
Tuesday 26th	300	350
Wednesday 27th	300	330
Thursday 28th	350	350
Friday 29th	330	270
Saturday 30th	320	300
Sunday 31st	350	320
Monday 1st	250	250
Tuesday 2nd	300	290
Wednesday 3rd	250	340
Thursday 4th	280	250

Figure 3.5 An example of how peak flow readings can be recorded without using graphs.

How do peak flow readings help diagnose asthma?

One of the ways asthma is diagnosed is to try asthma treatment in a person with symptoms suggesting the condition. Then there are two ways to tell if this treatment is working. The first is to ask the person if they feel better; the second is to do lung function tests, which is a more reliable way to find out whether the person has improved and, if so, by how much.

- If anti-asthma medication makes you better, you may have asthma – sometimes this medicine needs to be continued for quite a few weeks, or even months, before it starts to work.

- If the peak expiratory flow improves with treatment, this helps to confirm the diagnosis of asthma.

On a peak flow chart used to diagnose asthma, there are three things to watch for to see if there are any improvements:

- an increase in the readings (this should be at least 20% for the diagnosis to be confirmed)

- a decreased gap between the morning and evening readings

- a great reduction in early morning dips in the readings.

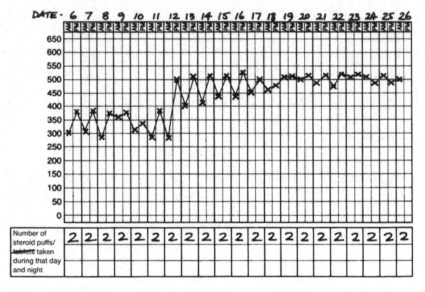

Figure 3.6 Peak flow chart showing a gradual improvement in readings after starting inhaler treatment for asthma.

Figure 3.6 shows two of these things. This man saw his doctor who suspected asthma from the medical history, and started treatment with an inhaled steroid (anti-asthma treatment) at two puffs twice a day. The man was asked to keep a record of his morning and evening peak flow readings. The graph shows the improvement in readings, which gradually increase from 300 to around 500. Also, the gap between the morning and evening readings gets less during the following weeks and the readings level off after about 4 weeks. This chart has confirmed that the man got better with the treatment and the diagnosis is asthma.

Is it really asthma, and is there more than one type?

My doctor has diagnosed 'viral-associated wheeze' in my 3-year-old son. What does he mean by that – I thought he had asthma?

You have probably mentioned to your doctor that your son's wheezing is triggered by colds. It is quite normal for young children under 5 years old to have about six or seven colds every year, but in some children the cold virus sets off chest symptoms, one of which is wheezing.

Viral-associated wheeze (also referred to as VAW by some doctors) is wheezing that is triggered only by viral infections. Specialists are not sure if wheezing that happens with virus infections is a type of asthma.

What you tell your doctor about your son's wheezing will help him to diagnose the cause of your son's wheezing and to decide on the right treatment. The cause of his wheezing may be due to asthma if there is a family member who has asthma. Another clue that he may have asthma is if your son has had *eczema* in the past or any other allergies.

When children who have asthma get a virus infection, their symptoms persist longer than in children without asthma. This may have something to do with their ability to fight infection.

Viral wheezing often improves with age, and in some children goes away altogether. If your child has eczema and there is a family history of asthma, the wheezing may continue, and this will make an asthma diagnosis more likely. Having parents who smoke is another important factor that increases the chance that a wheezy child has asthma. If you (and/or your partner) smoke, stopping smoking will really benefit you, your son and others around you.

Although your doctor has not confirmed the diagnosis of asthma in your son, asthma-reliever inhaler medicines are helpful in treating wheezing. If the viral wheezing is very bad and your son's breathing is difficult, doctors sometimes prescribe a short course of steroid tablets for a few days to get over the crisis period. Your son will also need an inhaler medicine (the reliever inhaler, usually coloured blue) to 'open up' and relax the airways, so that air can get in and out more easily when he breathes.

Unfortunately, asthma can be difficult to diagnose in this age group, mainly because it is difficult to get them to do blowing tests. If your son continues to wheeze with colds, simple blowing tests with a peak flow meter will help to confirm the diagnosis of asthma when he is about 6 years of age.

What other diseases can be incorrectly diagnosed instead of asthma?

Are there any ailments or illnesses associated with asthma?

Yes – there are three common and very important conditions that are closely associated with asthma:

- *eczema*

- *allergic rhinitis* (e.g. hay fever due to grass pollen, allergy to house dust mites)

- a general allergy to various things (e.g. cats, dogs, horses, house dust mite and some medicines).

Another very important condition in adults, which may be difficult to distinguish from asthma, is *chronic obstructive pulmonary disease* (COPD). In COPD, lung function tests such as *spirometry* do not usually improve, as they do in people with asthma. The two conditions may occur together, particularly in older people. It can sometimes be difficult to tell the difference between asthma and COPD, especially in people with very severe chronic (ongoing) asthma. In these people the spirometry tests may be similar to those in people with COPD. This condition is called 'chronic asthma with fixed airflow limitation'.

There are other conditions that are less common but also related to asthma, including *polyps* (small non-cancerous growths) in the nose and allergic skin conditions such as *urticaria*. Urticaria consists of raised blotchy patches on the skin looking very much like nettle rash.

How does asthma differ from chest conditions and other breathing difficulties?

Asthma is a condition in which symptoms are caused by narrowing of the airways that is reversible or variable, as described earlier in this chapter. This means that symptoms come and go, and for much of the time people with asthma are completely well. For example, athletes with asthma are able to perform at their peak when their asthma is well controlled. This is the main difference between asthma and other chest conditions.

Personal asthma action plan – things you might wish to discuss with your doctor or nurse once the possibility of asthma has been diagnosed.

If you think you or your child may have asthma, there are a number of questions to ask your doctor or nurse:

- Are my/my child's symptoms due to asthma?

- How can the diagnosis be confirmed?

- Shall I keep a peak flow chart over a few weeks?

- Is it worth trying asthma medication to see if this helps my/my child's symptoms?

If your doctor or nurse has confirmed a diagnosis of asthma in you or your child, you might want to ask about the treatments available:

- What are the options for me/my child?

- Which type of inhaler device is best for me/my child?

People with newly diagnosed asthma will benefit from having a personalised action plan – ask your doctor or asthma nurse for one.

Do look at the internet for more information. Some useful, reliable sites are listed at the end of this book.

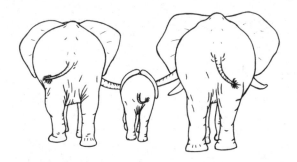

4 | Treatments for asthma

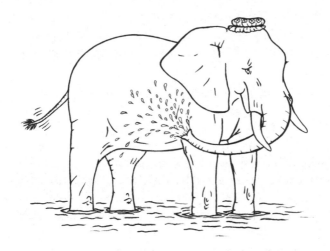

In this chapter you will learn about:

- the effect of reducing exposure to asthma triggers

- why asthma goes out of control and symptoms flare up

- the different medicines that are used to treat asthma

- the different inhaler devices that are available

- how to alter your medicines to help control your asthma.

NON-MEDICINE TREATMENTS

Allergen avoidance

People who have been exposed to certain *allergens* may get *allergic reactions* when they come into contact with them again. It makes sense for people to avoid the allergens that trigger their asthma.

Will complete allergen avoidance cure my asthma?

Complete avoidance is very rarely possible but, when it is, the asthma may improve. However, asthma is often caused by many things, of which allergy is only one. A complete cure is seen mainly in people who are exposed and become *sensitised* to their trigger allergens only at work (*occupational asthma*); when they change to a job where they are no longer exposed, their condition is 'cured'.

Even if it won't cure my asthma, would it help the asthma if I completely avoid exposure to allergens?

That depends on the allergens and how frequently and how much you are exposed. Sometimes complete avoidance reduces asthma symptoms but, in many cases, it does not.

Will reducing my exposure to trigger allergens improve my symptoms?

Yes, this is possible. Unfortunately, it is not always the case. Research has shown that reducing exposure only to *house dust mite* in the home is unlikely to reduce asthma symptoms. This is also true for other *allergens*. Still, most allergy specialists advise people with asthma to try to reduce their exposure to as many allergens as possible, hoping that this will reduce the symptoms and make the asthma more stable.

In the light of this research, it is not possible to give firm recommendations on how far you should go in trying to avoid allergens that trigger your asthma. The effect should always be balanced against the efforts required – the expense and the impact that the measures have on your lifestyle.

There are a wide range of allergy-reducing products that can be purchased. The manufacturers of these products make great claims that getting rid of allergens (mainly the house dust mite) from the home environment improves asthma. Some of them may be effective in reducing the number of house dust mites but do not necessarily improve asthma symptoms. Nearly all of the products are expensive, so we strongly recommend that you get specialist advice before spending money and time in the hope of a miracle cure.

My child has been diagnosed as having asthma. Should we have the cat put to sleep (or rehomed)?

Having the cat put to sleep, or even rehomed, is a drastic solution to the problem, even if your child has a true allergy to cats. We recommend that you discuss the question carefully with your doctor or nurse. Removing a much-loved family pet sometimes causes so much emotional upset that the asthma may become worse for a while. If you decide to remove your cat, it will take several weeks before you can assess whether the asthma has got better, because the cat allergens will stay in the house for many weeks after its removal.

Some people find that their asthma improves after a pet is removed from the home; others do not. Some find that, after their cat has been removed, they get more severe asthma reactions when they are next exposed to cats.

The presence of a cat in the house may cause or worsen asthma or, on the other hand, protect the person from getting severe asthma reactions on exposure outside their home. The theory of how this works is similar to the way we are immunised to certain diseases by having vaccinations (e.g. against tetanus, polio and diphtheria). By being exposed to cat *dander* over a period of time, the body gets used to (or immune to) it.

Washing or wiping the cat with a damp cloth once or twice a week may reduce the amount of cat allergen on its fur, but has very little impact on asthma symptoms – and washing or wiping a cat is easier said than done!

What we have said here about cats may also be true for other pets.

MEDICINES

If your treatment is not named in the book, it does not mean that you are receiving an unacceptable medicine. It is just that, for reasons of space, we cannot include all possible medicine names in the answer to each question. An added complication is that each medicine has a minimum of two names! The *generic name* is the basic or chemical name, but each medicine also has a *brand name*, given by a particular manufacturer. For example, the most frequently prescribed medicine for asthma is salbutamol (generic name). This is best known by the brand name Ventolin given by its leading manufacturer, but also by other names such as Salamol, Airomir or Asmasal depending on the country where it is used or the company that markets it. We will refer generally to generic names, as these are always mentioned on the medication packaging, and many are simply prescribed by their generic names.

At present, inhaled asthma medicines are placed into one of two categories – *preventers* and *relievers*. Relievers are either short- or long-acting.

- **Preventer** (also called 'controller' or 'anti-inflammatory') **drugs** prevent asthma symptoms if they are taken every day. They are usually taken by being inhaled. Steroid medicines are the most effective type of preventers. There are many different steroid inhalers, such as beclometasone, fluticasone, budesonide, ciclesonide and mometasone (brand names include AeroBec, Alvesco, Asmanex, Becotide, Filair, Flixotide, Pulmicort and Qvar).

- **Short-acting reliever medicines** (also called 'rescue' medicines or 'short-acting beta-agonist bronchodilators' – SABAs) As the name suggests, these *bronchodilators* relieve symptoms when they occur and therefore are used when needed and should not have to be taken regularly. They work within minutes, reaching maximum benefit after 15–20 minutes, and the effect lasts for around 4 hours. If you need to use your reliever more than twice a week, you need to arrange to see your doctor or asthma nurse urgently.

- **Long-acting reliever medicines** (also called 'long-acting beta-agonist bronchodilators' – LABAs, or 'long-acting-antimuscarinic bronchodilators' – LAMAs) These bronchodilators are recommended for people who are already taking inhaled corticosteroids (steroids) but need additional treatment to control their asthma symptoms. LABAs, such as salmeterol (Serevent) and formoterol (Oxis, Foradil), work for up to 12 hours. They must be prescribed as one of two drugs in one inhaler, so that the LABA cannot be taken without the inhaled corticosteroid. Tiotropium Respimat® is licensed for severe asthma, together with the inhaled corticosteroid, and is used once daily.

All relievers work in the same way   by relaxing tight muscles in the lining of the airways.

Other medicines include the following.

- **Leukotriene receptor antagonists** (LRTAs). These are available as tablets for children aged 2 years and over, and as granules for children as young as 6 months old. They work as preventer medicines but are not as effective as steroid medicines. They are given mainly as additional treatment to inhaled steroid and long-acting reliever inhalers, if asthma symptoms persist. They may also be used in older children and adults with *allergic rhinitis* (such as hay fever) who are taking inhaled steroids for their asthma because they may have some effect in both asthma and rhinitis.

- **Combination treatments**. There are a number of combination treatments, using an inhaled steroid preventer medicine (such as budesonide, beclometasone, fluticasone) with a long-acting or short-acting reliever medicine (formoterol, salmeterol, salbutamol) in one inhaler. (Trade names include Fostair, Flutiform, Symbicort, Seretide and DuoResp Spiromax.)

Because long-acting reliever medicines (salmeterol, formoterol) should be given *only* to people with asthma who are already taking inhaled steroids, combination treatment is considered the preferred way to administer long-acting relievers. When the two drugs are given in separate inhalers, some people stop their inhaled steroid, which is really bad because trying to control asthma with long-acting reliever medicines alone may lead to very severe asthma attacks.

My doctor has mentioned prednisolone. What is it and what does it do?

Prednisolone is one of a group of medicines whose proper name is *corticosteroids* (but often referred to as 'steroids'). We do not completely understand all its actions in asthma. However, we do know that it dampens down inflammation dramatically and controls the production of phlegm.

Prednisolone is the most commonly prescribed *oral steroid* medicine. It is used to treat *acute* attacks of asthma and, much less commonly, as long-term therapy for people with *chronic* severe asthma. Sometimes people are given a course of prednisolone to use at home as set out in their personal action plan.

In an acute asthma attack, it is important that high-enough doses of prednisolone are prescribed, and that it is given for a long enough time for the inflammation to subside. In an adult such a dose would usually be in the range of 30–60 mg/day, and for a child 1–2 mg per kilogram weight per day (up to 40 mg a day).

There is a form of prednisolone that dissolves in water. This is useful for children, and for people who find tablets hard to swallow. Taking the prednisolone with food, rather than on an empty stomach, may also reduce the risk of indigestion associated with these medicines.

Why won't my GP prescribe antibiotics for me to have at home so that I can take them at the first sign of a chest infection? This form of treatment means less time off work for me, and less pressure from my employers, which tends to make my asthma worse.

This is a rather tricky question, which, without knowing your individual details, we will have to answer in general terms. The difficulty is that the symptoms of worsening asthma and a true chest infection may be similar. They share many signs and symptoms, such as coughing, wheezing, shortness of breath and coughing up lots of phlegm.

In people with asthma these symptoms are much more likely to be caused by the asthma than by a bacterial infection. Therefore, it is usually much better for you to increase your asthma medication at the start of these symptoms than to start with an antibiotic. If your symptoms do not improve, you need to consult your doctor or nurse to see if any other treatment is needed.

Although antibiotics may help to clear a chest infection rapidly, they are not normally helpful in the treatment of asthma. Although asthma is often triggered by an infection, such as the common cold, this infection is nearly always caused by a virus. Viruses are not affected at all by antibiotics, so there is no point giving them to treat virus infections.

Should I have an anti-flu injection?

Routine influenza vaccination of children and adults with asthma is recommended.

Virus infections are important triggers of asthma in many people. Influenza (better known as 'flu') is a particularly important virus infection. It can result in serious pneumonia, particularly in older people or those with chronic chest trouble. For these people with asthma, flu may bring on a severe episode of asthma. So it is generally recommended that they have an anti-flu injection once a year, which may help to prevent the illness or at least reduce its severity.

There are few side-effects from this injection. Some people may suffer from a mild flu-like illness for a few days after the injection and a little soreness at the injection site.

Devices

Inhaler devices are used to get medicines directly into the lungs. This is the safest and best way to take asthma medicines, mainly because lower doses can be used and therefore with fewer side-effects than tablets.

There are many different inhaler devices for using asthma medicines. They can be divided into:

- pressurised metered-dose inhalers (pMDIs)
- *breath-activated* pressurised inhalers
- dry-powder inhalers
- spacer devices
- Soft-Mist inhalers (used in very severe asthma)
- nebulisers.

Pressurised metered-dose inhalers

These are sometimes called 'press and breathe' inhalers. They use a special sort of harmless gas to help release the treatments for asthma.

Many people use pressurised metered-dose inhalers (pMDIs) for their asthma but, sadly, don't always know how to use them correctly. There are a number of devices available for teaching people how to use their inhaler. One of these is the Trainhaler (see Figure 4.2). This 'dummy' inhaler comes with a Flotone, which is a small spacer device with a whistle that fits on the end of a pMDI. The whistle provides a signal when the person breathes in (inhales) at the correct speed. With the person inhaling through the Flotone, the whistle sounds when the correct flow is achieved, signalling when to

HOW TO USE A METERED-DOSE INHALER

1. Remove the cap.

2. Shake the inhaler.

3. Breathe out as far as is comfortable.

4. Hold the inhaler upright with your thumb on the base, below the mouthpiece. Place the mouthpiece in your mouth, between your teeth, and close your lips round it. Do not bite it.

5. Breathe in through your mouth. Just after starting to breathe in, press down on the top of the canister to release a puff of medicine. Continue to breathe in slowly for 5 seconds.

6. Hold your breath for 10 seconds or as long as possible, and then breathe out slowly.

7. Wait for a few seconds before repeating steps 2–6.

8. Replace the cap.

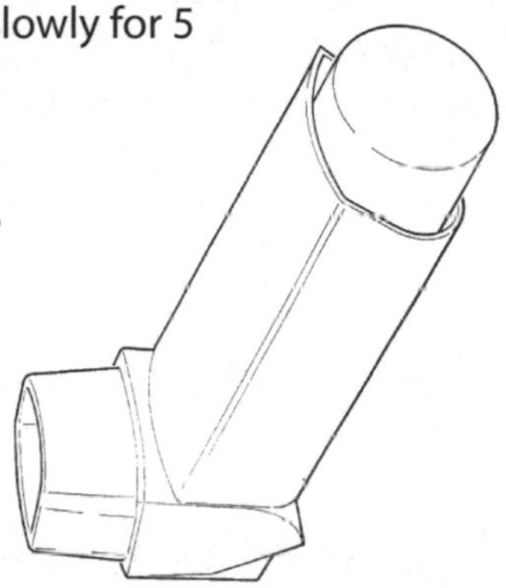

YOU SHOULD ALWAYS BE SHOWN HOW TO USE THE DEVICE

Figure 4.1 How to use the pressurised metered-dose inhaler (pMDI).

Just after starting to breathe in slowly, press the canister and continue to breathe in slowly: take 5 seconds to ensure that you breathe in long enough for the medicine to reach your lungs.

© Education for Health; adapted with permission from Education for Health, Warwick (www.educationforhealth.org)

press the inhaler to activate it. Then, as long as the person continues to breathe at the correct speed, the whistle continues.

Breath-activated pressurised devices

There are currently four breath-activated devices:

- the Autohaler
- the Easi-Breathe
- the Novoliser
- the Spiromax.

The medicine is contained in canisters, like the pressurised metered-dose inhaler, but the dose of medicine is not released until you breathe in. These devices are easier to use than the metered-dose inhaler because they do not rely on good hand–breath coordination. See Figures 4.3 and 4.4 on how to use these devices.

Dry-powder inhalers

Dry-powder inhalers are available as either single-dose or reservoir devices.

Single-dose dry-powder inhalers

Examples of single-dose dry-powder inhalers include the Diskus/ Accuhaler, the Aerolizer and the Diskhaler.

The **Diskus/Accuhaler** contains 60 doses of medicine enclosed in a foil strip within the inhaler. Each dose is separately sealed and is not exposed until the lever is set (see Figure 4.5).

The **Aerolizer** uses capsules that are loaded into the device. Holes are pricked at each end of the capsule before the medicine is inhaled (see Figure 4.6).

HOW TO USE THE TRAINHALER

1. Hold the device upright with your thumb on the base, below the mouthpiece.

2. Breathe out as far as is comfortable (don't breathe in again yet).

3. Place the device between your teeth, but do not bite it.

4. Close your lips around the device.

5. Breathe in gently through your mouth.

6. When you hear the device whistle, press down on the top of the canister. You will hear a sound like a puff of aerosol.

7. Continue to breathe in steadily and deeply, keeping the whistle going for as long as you can (5 seconds).

8. Hold your breath and remove the device from your mouth.

9. Continue holding your breath for as long as is comfortable. Then breathe normally.

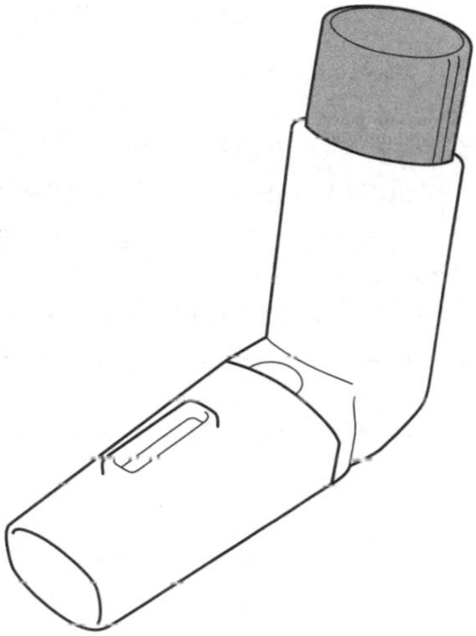

YOU SHOULD ALWAYS BE SHOWN HOW TO USE THE DEVICE

Figure 4.2 The Trainhaler – one of the devices used to help people learn how to use their inhaler correctly and effectively.

© Education for Health; adapted with permission from Education for Health, Warwick (www.educationforhealth.org)

HOW TO USE THE AUTOHALER

1. Remove the cap by pulling down on the tiny lip at the back.

2. Shake the inhaler.

3. Hold the inhaler upright and push the red lever up.

4. Breathe out gently. Keeping the inhaler upright, seal your lips firmly round the mouthpiece. Do not block the air vents on the bottom of the device.

5. Breathe in steadily and deeply through your mouth. DON'T stop breathing when the inhaler 'clicks' but continue taking this single really deep breath.

6. Hold your breath for about 10 seconds. Breathe out gently. Push the red lever down.

7. If a second dose is needed, wait several seconds before repeating steps 2–6.

8. If this is a brand new Autohaler, or if it has not been used for 48 hours, it should be primed before use (see step 9).

9. *To prime the device:* Raise the red lever. Press the white test-fire slide on the bottom of the inhaler in the direction of the arrow. Press the lever down. Repeat step 9 once more for two priming sprays.

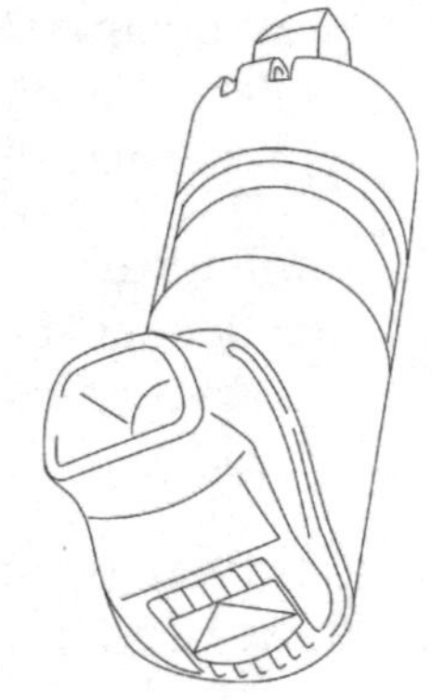

YOU SHOULD ALWAYS BE SHOWN HOW TO USE THE DEVICE

Figure 4.3 How to use the Autohaler.

© Education for Health; adapted with permission from Education for Health, Warwick (www.educationforhealth.org)

HOW TO USE THE EASI-BREATHE

1. Shake the inhaler.

2. Hold the inhaler upright. Open the cap.

3. Breathe out gently. Hold the inhaler upright, put the mouthpiece in your mouth and close your lips and teeth round it. (Do not block the air holes with your hand.)

4. Breathe in steadily through the mouthpiece. DON'T stop breathing when the inhaler 'puffs' but continue taking a really deep breath.

5. Hold your breath for about 10 seconds.

6. After use, hold the inhaler upright and immediately close the cap.

7. For a second dose, wait a few seconds before repeating steps 1–6.

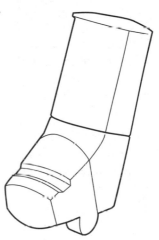

YOU SHOULD ALWAYS BE SHOWN HOW TO USE THE DEVICE

Figure 4.4 How to use the Easi-Breathe.

© Education for Health; adapted with permission from Education for Health, Warwick (www.educationforhealth.org)

HOW TO USE THE DISKUS/ACCUHALER

1. Open the device by holding the outer casing in one hand, while pushing the thumb grip away, until you hear a click.

2. Hold the device with the mouthpiece towards you; slide the lever away until it clicks. This makes the dose available for inhalation and moves the dose counter on.

3. Holding the device level, breathe out gently away from the device, put the mouthpiece in your mouth and take a breath in steadily and deeply.

4. Remove the device from your mouth and hold your breath for about 10 seconds

5. To close the device, slide the thumb grip back towards you as far as it will go until it clicks.

6. For a second dose, repeat steps 1–5.

7. The dose counter counts down from 60 to 0. The last five numbers are red.

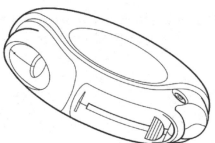

YOU SHOULD ALWAYS BE SHOWN HOW TO USE THE DEVICE

Figure 4.5 How to use the Diskus/Accuhaler.

© Education for Health; adapted with permission from Education for Health, Warwick (www.educationforhealth.org)

The **Diskhaler** uses foil disks that contain either four or eight individual doses of medicine. These disks are placed inside the device. The medicine is released by puncturing one of the doses on the disk which then allows you to breathe it in (see Figure 4.7).

Reservoir dry-powder devices

Examples of reservoir dry-powder devices include the Easyhaler, Clickhaler, Novolizer, Pulvinal, Turbohaler and Twisthaler.

The **Easyhaler** (Figure 4.8) is compact and releases one dose of medicine each time the top is pressed down. It has a number counter and a see-through window where the amount of powder present can be seen.

The **Clickhaler** (Figure 4.9) has a number counter and looks a little like a metered-dose inhaler. When the top is pressed to activate one dose, a clicking sound is heard – hence the name of the device. The slightly elongated mouthpiece is ideal for children who have fixed braces on their teeth, because they are able to seal their lips securely around the mouthpiece before breathing in the medicine.

The **Novolizer** (Figure 4.10) is a novel device with a replaceable medication cartridge. There is a number counter as well as a small window that changes from green to red following correct inhalation. This device makes a loud click sound when the person has inhaled the drug correctly.

Both the **Flexhaler** (Figure 4.11) and the **Pulvinal** (Figure 4.12) release one dose at a time when you twist the body of the inhaler. These devices have a see-through window to show how much medication is left.

The **Turbohaler** (or **Turbuhaler**) (Figure 4.13) also releases one dose at a time when the base is twisted. It contains either an indicator or a number counter, to help you to check how much medicine is left.

The **Twisthaler** (Figure 4.14) releases the medicine ready to breathe in when you take the inhaler top off. It also has a number counter, which locks once the last dose is used and prevents the inhaler from being used again.

HOW TO USE THE AEROLIZER

1. Remove the cap.

2. Hold the inhaler at the base and turn the mouthpiece in the direction of the arrow.

3. Place a capsule in the compartment in the base of the inhaler.

4. Twist the mouthpiece back to the closed position; you will hear a click.

5. Hold the inhaler upright, squeezing the two blue buttons on the base of inhaler inwards to pierce the capsule; then release them.

6. Breathe out gently.

7. Insert the mouthpiece into your mouth, sealing your lips and teeth around the mouthpiece.

8. Breathe in quickly and deeply. You should hear a rattling of the capsule.

9. Remove the inhaler from your mouth.

10. Hold your breath for a count of 10, or as long as is comfortable.

11. Breathe out gently.

12. Discard the capsule from the compartment in the base of the inhaler.

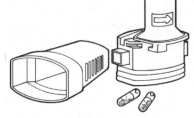

13. Replace the cap.

YOU SHOULD ALWAYS BE SHOWN HOW TO USE THE DEVICE

Figure 4.6 How to use the Aerolizer.

© Education for Health; adapted with permission from Education for Health, Warwick (www.educationforhealth.org)

HOW TO USE THE DISKHALER

1. To load a disk, remove the mouthpiece cover, pull the white tray out by squeezing the white ridges at either side and put the disk on top with the numbers uppermost

2. Replace the tray and rotate the disk in and out until the number 8 (or 4 if a 4-dose disk) shows in the window.

3. To use the device, keeping it horizontal, lift the rear of the lid up as far as it will go, piercing the top and the bottom of the blister, then close the lid.

4. Keeping the device level, breathe out deeply, close your mouth round the mouthpiece (taking care not to block the air holes at the side) and breathe in as deeply as possible.

5. Remove the Diskhaler from your mouth and hold your breath for about 10 seconds; then breathe out slowly

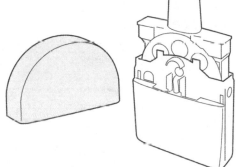

6. Slide the tray in and out ready for the next dose, then repeat steps 3–5

7. Replace the mouthpiece cover.

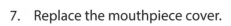

YOU SHOULD ALWAYS BE SHOWN HOW TO USE THE DEVICE

Figure 4.7 How to use the Diskhaler. It takes foil-covered disks containing either 4 or 8 measured doses, according to the prescription.

© Education for Health; adapted with permission from Education for Health, Warwick (www.educationforhealth.org)

HOW TO USE THE EASYHALER

1. Shake the device and then hold it upright.

2. Remove the mouthpiece cap.

3. Press the top of the device once. You will hear a click.

4. Breathe out normally and then place the mouthpiece between your teeth. Close your lips round the mouthpiece.

5. Take a strong and deep breath through the device. Hold your breath for 5–10 seconds and then breathe out away from the device.

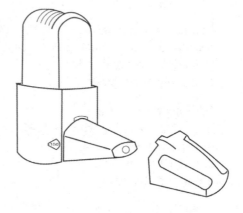

6. If you need to take another dose of inhaler medicine, repeat steps 3–5.

7. Replace the mouthpiece cap.

8. The counter on the side turns red when there are 20 doses left. When it shows zero (0), the device should be replaced.

YOU SHOULD ALWAYS BE SHOWN HOW TO USE THE DEVICE

Figure 4.8 How to use the Easyhaler.

© Education for Health; adapted with permission from Education for Health, Warwick (www.educationforhealth.org)

HOW TO USE THE CLICKHALER

1. Hold the device upright.

2. Remove the mouthpiece cover from the inhaler.

3. Shake the inhaler.

4. Continue to hold the inhaler upright with your thumb on the base and a finger on the coloured push (dosing) button.

5. Press the dosing button down firmly – once only – and then release.

6. Breathe out gently and then place the mouthpiece between your lips and teeth, sealing your lips round the mouthpiece. (Do not breathe out into the device.)

7. Breathe in steadily and deeply. Remove the device from your mouth and hold your breath for about 5–10 seconds. Breathe out slowly.

8. For a second dose, keep the device upright and repeat steps 3–7.

9. Replace the mouthpiece cover.

10. There is a dose counter at the back of the inhaler. After 190 doses a red warning appears in the counter window, which shows there are 10 doses left. When there are no doses left, the inhaler locks and can no longer be used, and should be discarded.

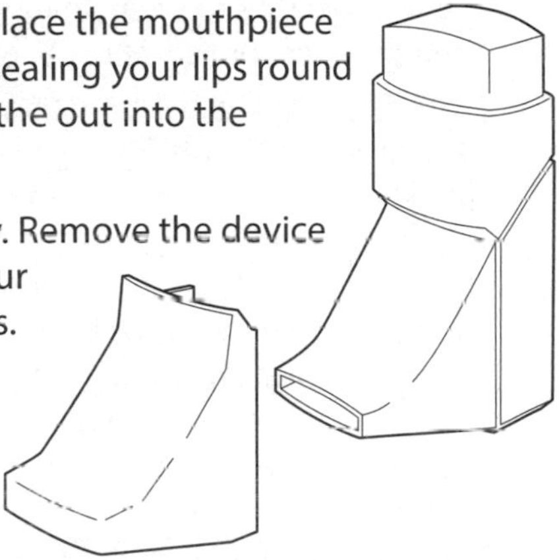

YOU SHOULD ALWAYS BE SHOWN HOW TO USE THE DEVICE

Figure 4.9 How to use the Clickhaler.

HOW TO USE THE NOVOLIZER

Inserting a cartridge into the device

1. On the top of the Novolizer device, remove the lid by squeezing both sides of the ribbed surface. Move the lid forwards and then lift off.
2. Insert the cartridge into the device with the dosage counter facing the mouthpiece.
3. Replace the lid using the lid guides. Push the lid down so that it is level with the button at the opposite end to the mouthpiece. It will click into place.

Using the device

1. Keeping the device level, remove the mouthpiece cap by squeezing the sides gently and sliding it forwards.
2. Press down the button at the back of the inhaler (at the opposite end to the mouthpiece) until you hear a click. The control window at the mouthpiece end of the device will change from red to green.
3. Breathe out before you place the inhaler device into your mouth. Do not breathe out through the device.
4. Put the mouthpiece into your mouth and breathe in fully and deeply through the device. You will hear a click if you breathe through the device correctly, and the control window will change from green to red. Hold your breath for a few seconds before taking the device out of your mouth and breathing out slowly
5. If a further dose is needed, repeat steps 2–4.
6. Replace the mouthpiece cap.
7. When the dose counter above the mouthpiece is on zero (0), the cartridge needs to be replaced.

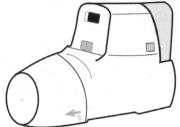

YOU SHOULD ALWAYS BE SHOWN HOW TO USE THE DEVICE

Figure 4.10 How to use the Novolizer

HOW TO USE THE FLEXHALER

1. Holding the device upright, unscrew and lift off the white cover.

2. To load the dose, hold the device upright with the mouthpiece on top, and twist the grip to the right and then back to the left until it clicks.

3. Do not shake the device.

4. Place the mouthpiece between your lips and teeth and breathe in (inhale) as forcefully and deeply as possible. (With the Patient Trainer *only*, a whistle sound indicates you've inhaled correctly.) Even when a full dose is taken, there may be no taste and no sensation of having inhaled any medication.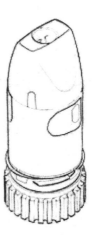

5. Remove the device from your mouth and hold your breath for about 10 seconds.

6. Breathe out – but **not** into the Flexhaler.

7. For a second dose, repeat steps 2–6.

8. The dose indicator window on the side of the device shows how many doses are left. When a zero (0) on the red background reaches the middle of the window, the Flexhaler should be discarded.

9. When using a brand new Flexhaler, prime it before using it the first time only. Twist the grip in one direction as far as it will go, then twist it fully back again in the other direction as far as it will go until it clicks.

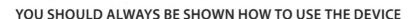

YOU SHOULD ALWAYS BE SHOWN HOW TO USE THE DEVICE

Figure 4.11 How to use the Flexhaler.

© Education for Health; adapted with permission from Education for Health, Warwick (www.educationforhealth.org)

HOW TO USE THE PULVINAL

1. Unscrew and take off the protective cover.

2. Hold the inhaler upright.

3. Press and hold the button on the mouthpiece.

4. Twist the base of the inhaler to the right, continuing to press the button until the red mark shows in the hole beneath the button.

5. Release the button on the mouthpiece and twist the inhaler back again in the opposite direction until it clicks and the red mark has changed to green.

6. Breathe out away from the mouthpiece, then put the inhaler mouthpiece between your lips and teeth.

7. Breathe in deeply and as quickly as possible.

8. Remove the inhaler from our mouth and hold your breath for about 10 seconds.

9. If other doses are required, repeat steps 2–8.

10. The amount of medication left in the device can be easily viewed through the clear wall of the device.

11. Replace the protective cover.

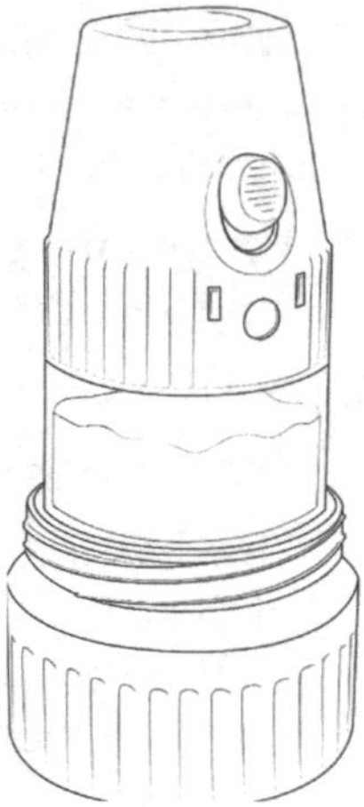

YOU SHOULD ALWAYS BE SHOWN HOW TO USE THE DEVICE

Figure 4.12 How to use the Pulvinal.

© Education for Health; adapted with permission from Education for Health, Warwick (www.educationforhealth.org)

HOW TO USE THE TURBOHALER/TURBUHALER

1. Unscrew and lift off the white cover.

2. Hold the main body of device upright and twist the (red) base as far as it will go, in both directions. You will hear a clicking sound.

3. Breathe out, away from the device mouthpiece.

4. Put the mouthpiece between your lips and teeth, and breathe in as deeply as possible.

5. Remove the device from your mouth and then breathe out.

6. For a second dose, repeat steps 2–5.

7. Replace the white cover.

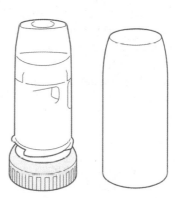

YOU SHOULD ALWAYS BE SHOWN HOW TO USE THE DEVICE

Figure 4.13 How to use the Turbohaler/Turbuhaler.

© Education for Health; adapted with permission from Education for Health, Warwick (www.educationforhealth.org)

Spacer devices

Spacer devices are 'holding chambers' and are used together with a pressurised metered-dose inhaler. The mouthpiece of the spacer is placed in the mouth and then the inhaler is used to spray the medicine into the spacer, which traps the medicine. This allows enough time for the medicine to be inhaled by normal breathing through the spacer mouthpiece. Children under the age of about 3 years will need to use a facemask instead of the mouthpiece attached to the spacer's mouthpiece.

Examples of spacers and spacers with masks and how to use them are shown in Figures 4.15 and 4.16.

Soft Mist Inhalers

This inhaler (called a Respimat®) is currently about the same size as a press and breathe inhaler and used with a drug called tiotropium, a long-acting reliever licensed for people with severe asthma. It acts similarly to a nebuliser in that the drug is converted into a fine mist which is easier to use compared with a pressurised metered dose inhaler.

Nebulisers

A **nebuliser** (Figure 4.17) is a device that can convert liquid medicine into a fine mist that can be inhaled easily by someone unable to use an inhaler. It is used in emergencies, either with oxygen or with room air.

HOW TO USE THE TWISTHALER

1. Hold the main body of the device, keeping it upright with the pink base at the bottom.

2. Unscrew the white cap counterclockwise and lift it off. Removing the cap loads the dose, and the counter will count down by one.

3. Check to be sure that the arrow is pointing towards the counter window.

4. Breathe out fully, away from the mouthpiece.

5. Holding the device level, put the mouthpiece between your lips and teeth. Seal your lips round the mouthpiece and take a deep, quick breath.

6. Remove the device from your mouth and hold your breath for about 10 seconds or as long as is comfortable. Breathe out, away from the mouthpiece.

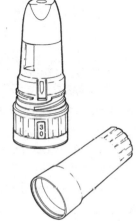

7. Then replace the cap, turning it clockwise until you hear a click.

8. If another dose is required, repeat steps 1–7.

9. Rinse your mouth after using the device.

10. The last dose is number 01.

11. The cap locks when the device is empty and the counter reads 00. Discard the device.

YOU SHOULD ALWAYS BE SHOWN HOW TO USE THE DEVICE

Figure 4.14 How to use the Twisthaler.

© Education for Health; adapted with permission from Education for Health, Warwick (www.educationforhealth.org)

HOW TO USE A SPACER

(Example shown is an Aerochamber)

Method for someone who can use the Aerochamber without help

1. Remove the caps of the metered-dose inhaler (MDI) and the spacer.
2. Shake the MDI and insert it into the back of the spacer.
3. Place the mouthpiece in your mouth; press the canister once to release one dose of medication.
4. Take a deep, slow breath in. If you hear a whistling sound, you are breathing in too quickly.
5. Hold your breath for about 10 seconds; then breathe out through the mouthpiece.

Method particularly useful for young children

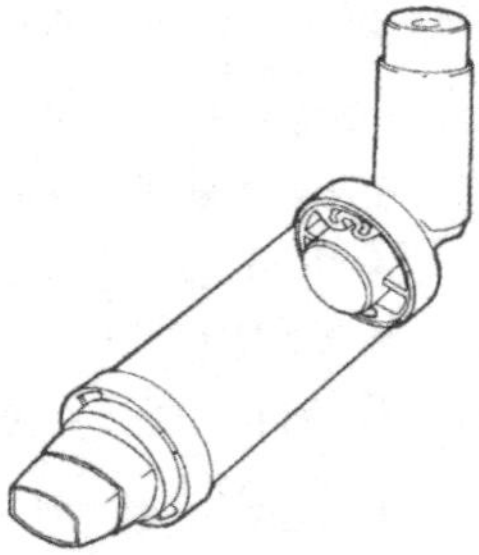

1. After removing the caps, shake the metered-dose inhaler (MDI) and insert it into the back of the spacer.
2. Place the mouthpiece in the child's mouth.
3. Encourage the child to breathe in and out, slowly and gently so that the device does not whistle.
4. Once the breathing pattern is well established, press the canister (once) to release one dose of medication. Leave the mouthpiece in position as the child continues to breathe in and out 5 more times.
5. Remove the spacer from the child's mouth.
6. For a second dose, wait a few seconds, and repeat steps 1–5.

YOU SHOULD ALWAYS BE SHOWN HOW TO USE THE DEVICE

Figure 4.15 How to use the Aerochamber spacer.

© Education for Health; adapted with permission from Education for Health, Warwick (www.educationforhealth.org)

HOW TO USE A SPACER WITH MASK

(Example shown is an Aerochamber with a mask)

1. Remove the caps of the metered-dose inhaler (MDI) device and the spacer.

2. Shake the MDI before each use.

3. Insert the MDI into the back of the spacer.

4. Apply the mask to your face and ensure there is a good seal.

5. Press the MDI once at beginning of slow breath in (inhalation). Maintain the seal for six (6) breaths.

6. Administer one puff at a time.

7. To clean the device, remove the back piece of the spacer. Soak the back piece and the rest of the device in lukewarm water and liquid detergent. Agitate gently but do not rinse. Allow to air dry in vertical position. Replace the back piece when the unit is completely dry.

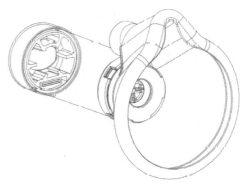

YOU SHOULD ALWAYS BE SHOWN HOW TO USE THE DEVICE

Figure 4.16 How to use a spacer with a mask.

© Education for Health; adapted with permission from Education for Health, Warwick (www.educationforhealth.org)

HOW TO USE A NEBULISER*

1. Clean and/or disinfect the nebuliser before using it.
2. Remove the top of the nebuliser by twisting it counterclockwise.
3. Pour the prescribed medication into the nebuliser cup.
4. Replace the top of the nebuliser.
5. If using a mask, attach it directly to the nebuliser outlet.
6. If using a mouthpiece, attach it so that the blue valve is facing up.
7. Connect the tubing to the air intake at the bottom of the nebuliser cup.
8. Sit in a relaxed, upright position and turn on the air compressor.
9. Close your lips round mouthpiece, placing the mouthpiece on top of your tongue and inhale the aerosol mist slowly through your mouth.
10. If using a mask, place the mask over your mouth and nose, and inhale the aerosol mist slowly.
11. Exhale slowly.
12. Continue steps 9 – 11 until the medication is gone or you hear a sputtering sound.
13. Turn off the air compressor.
14. Disconnect the tubing from the bottom of the nebuliser air intake.
15. Disassemble the nebuliser and follow the printed instructions for cleaning and disinfecting.

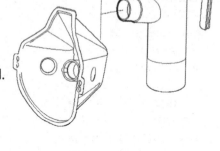

YOU SHOULD ALWAYS BE SHOWN HOW TO USE A NEBULISER

Figure 4.17 How to use a nebuliser.

*Pari LC Plus nebulizer

© Education for Health; adapted with permission from Education for Health, Warwick (www.educationforhealth.org)

Is it safe to use more than the stated dose of my reliever (blue) inhaler?

Your blue inhaler contains either salbutamol (e.g. Ventolin) or terbutaline (Bricanyl). It is a reliever, works within a few minutes and is usually very effective. It contains medicines that relax the tightness in the muscles in your airways.

It won't hurt you to take more in the short term, but the important thing is to know why you need to take more than the stated dose. It is normally a danger sign indicating that your asthma is getting worse or poorly controlled. Therefore, your blue inhaler becomes less effective and relieves your 'tightness' for only a very short time. It may be tempting to keep on taking puffs of your reliever (even though it doesn't seem to be doing much good) but this can be dangerous. If it is not having its usual effect, you should seek urgent medical help.

Once your airways have become very inflamed and narrow, salbutamol or terbutaline has little effect. Other medicines such as steroid inhaler or tablets will be needed to treat your asthma, and you may have to take a regular steroid inhaler medicine as well as other treatments.

I don't want to become dependent on my inhalers. Will this happen if I take them regularly?

You won't become dependent on your asthma inhalers. The reliever inhalers (e.g. salbutamol Ventolin; or terbutaline, Bricanyl) should be taken on an 'as required' basis rather than regularly. These drugs work for about 4 hours and are designed to give instant relief when your air passages are tight. They don't provide long-term benefit. If you need to take your reliever more than twice a week your asthma is out of control and you should see your doctor urgently. You may need regular preventer treatment or an adjustment of the preventer treatment you already take. Nowadays it is thought best to take preventer treatment if a reliever medicine is needed more than twice a week.

The preventer medicines (e.g. the inhaled steroids, AeroBec, Alvesco, Asmabec, Asmanex, Becotide, Flixotide, Pulmicort, Pulvinal [beclometasone], Qvar) do not give immediate relief. Therefore, you need to take them regularly, as prescribed by your doctor, for long periods of time. Preventer medicines will control the inflammation in the airways; they are not addictive and you will not become dependent on them.

Are there any side-effects from inhaled steroids?

When taken in low doses the most common side-effect of *inhaled (topical) corticosteroids is* hoarseness (huskiness) of the voice but very few people are affected in this way. When this occurs, it may be reduced by gargling or rinsing out the mouth after using the inhaler. It disappears if the treatment is stopped. Hoarseness is seen more often in people who use their voice (singers, teachers etc.).

Another problem can be *thrush* of the mouth (also known as candida infection), where the back of the throat becomes sore and is red with white spots and an unpleasant taste. This may be prevented by using your inhaler before brushing your teeth or just before you eat or by rinsing your mouth out very well after the inhalation. You can also prevent or reduce it by using a spacer device (see Figures 4.15 and 4.16).

Both hoarseness and thrush are more likely to occur the more often the inhaled steroid medicines are taken (once, twice or three times a day) or when high doses are needed to control your asthma.

One of the inhaled steroid medicines called ciclesonide (Alvesco) is inactive in the mouth and works only when it reaches the lungs. So this medicine is less likely to cause oral thrush, and may be chosen by a doctor for someone affected this way.

Children taking regular inhaled steroids are much less likely than adults to develop thrush or hoarseness.

If **high doses** of steroid inhalers are used over many years, there may be an increased risk of thinning of the bones (*osteoporosis*) so that they become weaker and fracture more easily. However, this risk from long-term use of steroid inhalers is much less serious than the risks of asthma that is not well controlled or from the frequent use of steroid tablets, which may weaken your bones and increase your risk of fractures to a much greater extent.

Will the steroids stunt my child's growth?

Occasional short courses of oral steroids, such as prednisolone, will not affect your child's growth even when they are given in high doses. They are essential in the management of an acute asthma attack, and can be life-saving. If these short courses are required several times each year, or if steroid tablets have to be taken over a long period of time (e.g. for months or years), they can reduce your child's growth – but so can poorly controlled asthma.

Research has been carried out on the effects of long-term inhaled steroid medicines and children's growth. Contrary to many worries, growth was found *not* to be adversely affected by steroid inhalers in doses that controlled the asthma of the vast majority of children. Some children who require higher doses of inhaled steroids (400 micrograms (μg) or more per day) grow less well during the first year of treatment, after which they grow at a normal rate.

A balance must be drawn between the known effect of uncontrolled asthma in reducing children's growth and the possible effect of high-dose inhaled steroids in doing the same. If high doses of inhaled steroid are needed, your child should be under the care of a children's doctor (paediatrician) who specialises in asthma.

Will the steroids weaken my child's bones?

Occasional short courses of oral steroids, such as prednisolone, do not have any weakening effect on your child's bones. There is no risk of bone fractures in people taking *inhaled* corticosteroids. However, if your child needs more than two or three courses per year of steroid *tablets*, that may weaken the child's bones and increase the risk of a fracture. Therefore it is very important that your child regularly takes the medication advised by your doctor – in order to prevent asthma attacks and therefore reduce the need for corticosteroid tablets. Therefore, regular preventer treatment with inhaled steroids is better for your child's bones than taking a couple of courses of oral steroid tablets every year.

Why do I keep getting white spots on the back of my throat?

It is likely that you have thrush infection in your throat. This is also known as 'candida' or 'monilia' infection, but is best known as *thrush*. It is a fungus infection, and is one of the very few side-effects caused by inhaled steroids. Read more about this in the answer about possible side-effects of inhaled steroids.

I read in the paper that asthma treatments are dangerous. Is this true?

No. The treatments are not dangerous but asthma itself can be dangerous if it is not controlled. In low doses there are no serious side-effects from any of the asthma medicines. If the doses are increased, the risks of side-effects are greater. However, doses are increased only when asthma is not controlled or is getting worse, so people will always be more at more risk from the asthma itself than from the treatment required to control it.

Very rarely, high doses of inhaled steroids over long periods of time and steroid tablets may affect the body's normal reaction to severe stress, such as an infection or surgery, by dampening the body's normal response to these incidents by suppressing the action of the *adrenal* glands. This may lead to a collapse with a fall in blood pressure and low levels of sugar in the blood. Such cases require acute medical interventions. Other potential side-effects of steroids are discussed in the answer about side-effects of inhaled steroids.

Theophylline medicines (*aminophylline*, Nuelin, Slo-Phyllin, Uniphyllin) are used less often now because other, newer, medicines are more effective. However, when they are used they may be dangerous if the levels in the blood are too high. Anyone taking these medicines should have a blood test from time to time to check that the levels are satisfactory. Some medicines, such as cimetidine (used for gastric acidity, Tagamet) or erythromycin (an antibiotic), increase the risk of problems with theophyllines. Always check with your doctor or asthma nurse if you are prescribed these medicines.

Make sure that you have a regular review with your doctor or asthma nurse. This may need to be only once or twice a year if all is going well. However, if your symptoms are worsening, you might need additional asthma medicines or to increase your existing treatments. Generally, the aim is for you to control your asthma with the lowest possible dose of a medicine. This is covered in Chapter 5, 'Beating asthma'.

Will steroids affect my teenage daughter's growth?

If your daughter takes *inhaled* steroids, this is most unlikely. The small effects that inhaled steroids may have on growth are mainly seen in children aged 6–9 years. However, if she takes high daily doses (800 micrograms (µg) or more) there may be a small reduction in her growth during the first year of treatment. If she is already taking inhaled steroids, it is unlikely that her growth will continue to be affected.

If she takes steroid *tablets* for a long time (months), growth can be temporarily reduced. There are extremely few children who require long-term corticosteroid tablets – provided they take their inhaled steroid as prescribed. So if she needs oral steroids, she may not be taking her inhaled steroid as she is supposed to. Check when she got the last prescription: if it is a long time ago, she is not taking it as regularly as she should.

Many children with asthma have a somewhat different growth pattern during puberty, and their adolescent growth spurt is somewhat stunted. These children normally continue to grow for longer periods than their peers, so they eventually reach a normal adult height but a couple of years later than their peers.

Can inhaled steroids make children hyperactive and cause sleep problems?

That is most unlikely. However, sometimes children become much more active when their asthma is controlled by the inhaled steroids. Some parents mistakenly interpret that as a side-effect. However, it merely reflects that the improved asthma control leads to a better night's sleep and gives the child more energy – their activity goes from reduced to normal.

Steroid tablets taken in high doses can cause side-effects such as mood changes, nightmares, mental disturbances and hyperactivity.

A few cases of unusual mood changes in people (both adults and children) taking beclometasone (Becotide) have been reported, but it does not necessarily mean that they were caused by the medicine.

I am really worried about my son, who has just been diagnosed with asthma. The specialist at the hospital wants to put him on Flixotide but the leaflet inside the packet says it's for children over the age of 4. He's only 2.

We understand your concerns about your son, especially if you have just found out that he has asthma. The good thing is that he is being seen by a hospital specialist who will have made sure that there is nothing else wrong with him.

Treatment for asthma at that age usually includes an inhaled steroid medicine, which will help to control his asthma. Medicines such as Flixotide are sometimes used 'off-label' in younger children. In your son's case it means that, when the medicine was licensed by the medicine safety authorities, research studies had not been carried out in children under 4 years of age. The product licence for this medicine could therefore only state that it was for use in children 4 years old or older; it does not mean that the medicine is unsafe or does not work in younger children. Do discuss with your doctor.

Licensing of medicines is based on research into the use of the drugs in humans. Carrying out research in children and pregnant women is always difficult because there are ethical and practical issues to be considered. For example, a child cannot give consent to be a test case for trying out a new medicine, and many parents are reluctant to take that decision for them. Similarly, pregnant women are unwilling to be used to test new medicines in case it affects the baby. This is why many drugs are said to be not suitable for (or haven't been tested in) children or pregnant women).

The specialist will be aware of the recommended age for using Flixotide and will have thought very carefully about the medicines needed to improve your son's asthma. The important thing is that your son is on preventer asthma treatment, which gives the best conditions for controlling his symptoms.

I have read on the internet that there is an injection treatment for allergic asthma called Xolair. Is this correct, and would it be useful for my child who has allergic asthma?

You are right, there is an injection treatment called omallzumab (Xolair). It is used to treat allergic asthma but only for those with moderate to severe asthma not controlled with high doses of inhaled steroid medication. It is not a substitute for the usual asthma treatments but it may allow lower doses of these drugs to be used to improve the asthma control or reduce the number of asthma flare-ups.

Xolair is an anti-immunoglobulin E (IgE) treatment. In allergy-triggered asthma, the body's IgE production is part of the allergic inflammatory process, which causes respiratory symptoms.

This injection treatment blocks IgE and prevents the inflammation from developing and the symptoms of asthma occurring. The treatment is very expensive and is reserved for adults and children over 12 years of age with severe allergic asthma that cannot be controlled by normal asthma treatments. The injection is given every two or four weeks. In most countries it can be prescribed only by respiratory specialist doctors.

Personal action plan – things you might wish to discuss with your doctor or nurse

It is important to make sure that you are on the right medication to control your asthma. It is possible that your asthma is perfectly controlled but, if not, you may need a higher or lower dose, or you may need a different kind of inhaler device.

At your next asthma review, ask whether your medication needs to be changed or adjusted. The following information will help the doctor to answer your questions. When your asthma is worse, tell the doctor or asthma nurse:

- what sort of symptoms you are having, particularly at night or when you exercise

- what inhaler medicines you are taking, and how often

- how much your asthma is troubling you

- if you have a problem

- what your peak flow readings (blowing tests) are like, and

- what your peak flow chart is like.

It is very helpful if you do a peak flow chart for the week or two before you go for your check-up, and take the chart with you.

5 | Controlling asthma

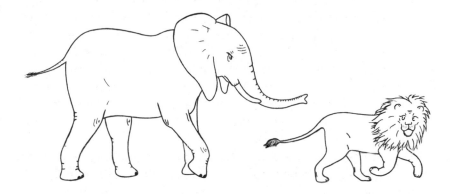

In this chapter you will learn:

- why asthma doesn't have to control your life
- how asthma can be controlled
- how to keep a check on your asthma (monitoring control)
- when to monitor your asthma
- what the warning signs are when asthma is out of control
- how you can help yourself
- when to call for help.

Success in looking after your asthma depends on knowing what is meant by good and poor asthma control. If you can tell when your asthma is well or poorly controlled, you can make changes to your treatment in response to changes in your symptoms. Getting the treatment right in the first place is a result of the partnership between you and your doctor, your nurse and other health professionals who may be involved in helping you to manage your asthma. Once you have been prescribed treatment, you are the person who needs to live with your asthma and recognise when symptoms change.

We believe that the best ways to monitor asthma are to use symptoms *and* peak expiratory flow readings (if you are able to use a peak flow meter). Peak flow readings are sometimes referred to as 'Lung Function tests' or 'blowing tests' but in this chapter we will use the term 'peak flow readings'. Peak flow meters can be prescribed by a doctor or can be bought over the counter (without a prescription). All peak flow meters give slightly different results; so it is best to have your own. If you can, take it with you when you go for an asthma check-up with your nurse or doctor.

There are many people with peak flow meters who take their readings only occasionally because they find it inconvenient to measure it every day. Although this is better than not recording them at all, regular measurements provide valuable information because peak flow readings often change before there are obvious symptoms of uncontrolled asthma. If you cannot or don't want to do your peak flow readings every day, perhaps record them when you have a cold or when you have asthma symptoms. These readings will help you decide whether and, if so, what extra asthma treatment you need and when to seek help. Your nurse, doctor or asthma 'educator' can help you to understand when to worry about your peak flow readings and when it is safe to continue to manage on your own. This information can be written down in a personal asthma action plan for you to look at when you need to check what you should do.

Many asthma attacks and admissions to hospital can be prevented by prompt action with the right treatment, provided that the attack is recognised early. We believe that helping you to recognise *uncontrolled asthma* is one of the most important functions of this book. Uncontrolled asthma means danger, and we urge you to read this section carefully.

One of the biggest changes in asthma care has been the introduction of action plans for all people with the condition. They are sometimes known as self-management plans because that's what they are for – to help you manage your asthma yourself. A personal asthma action plan provides you with information on how to check (or monitor) your asthma, how to tell if it is going out of control and what to do when this happens. These plans can vary from being a simple list of your asthma medicines and when to take them, to more detailed information, using peak flow readings with advice on when to start taking a course of steroid tablets for an attack. We know that such a plan can help you look after your asthma: the advice from experts around the world is that all people with the condition should have one!

My asthma nurse said that I must take responsibility for looking after myself and my asthma. What did she mean?

We all have some responsibilities to ourselves and our health. If you have asthma, learning about the illness is very helpful. You need to learn how it is treated and when to call for help. Although many children apparently 'grow out of' their asthma, it is a condition that often stays for life. There may be times, sometimes lasting several years, when it doesn't cause any problems; in such instances we say that the asthma has gone into *remission*. Unfortunately, symptoms can return or flare up, and it is helpful to be able to recognise this. As with many other situations in life, knowing what to do to when things go wrong will help you to be in control.

The main things you can do are to:

- avoid triggers that make your asthma worse

- take your medication as advised, and learn how to use the inhaler

- see your doctor or asthma nurse for regular check-ups

- learn how to recognise when your asthma is going out of control and what to do if that happens.

Many of these things are discussed in this chapter; the rest can be found in other sections of this book.

What can I do myself?

Probably the most important thing you can do is keep yourself fit and well: 20–30 minutes of brisk walking every day, or other forms of exercise, will help to keep you fit. Eating sensibly with a good, healthy, balanced diet is also essential; it should include some fruit and fresh vegetables every day. If you smoke, stopping smoking will be of enormous benefit to you both now and in the future. Smoke irritates the airways, stops your asthma medicines working well, increases respiratory illnesses in young children, causes lung cancer and other chest problems, and is generally antisocial. It is also expensive!

It may seem very obvious to say this but, if you have been prescribed medicines for your asthma, it is best to take them. We frequently meet patients who have had an asthma attack because they have stopped taking or run out of their asthma medicines. This is as frustrating for the health professionals as for the sufferers, because good control can be achieved when asthma medicines are taken regularly.

Asthma is a lifelong condition and most doctors and nurses will set up a system to help you obtain repeat prescriptions of your medicines, as well as an emergency supply of prednisolone (cortisone) tablets in case of asthma attacks. Your responsibility (or your carer's responsibility) is to make sure that the repeat prescription is ordered *before* the medicines run out.

Repeat prescription systems vary from practice to practice, but they do have a few things in common. There are usually a set number of repeat prescriptions (repeats) that can be authorised by the practice before you need to see the doctor or asthma nurse for a check-up. This is usually set for 3–12 repeats, depending on how often you have asthma symptoms and how severe your asthma is.

Regular check-ups either at the doctor's surgery or in a dedicated asthma clinic give you the opportunity to discuss your condition and to learn how you can recognise episodes when it is out of control. You can also learn how to deal with these episodes.

My doctor says I would benefit from attending his asthma clinic. What is this and what happens there?

General practitioners (GPs, family doctors) may provide a range of clinics where particular conditions (such as asthma or diabetes) or particular problems (such as stopping smoking or preventing heart disease) are dealt with in a specific clinic. Some of them are run by the GP, whilst others are run by the practice nurse. In some cases the GP and the asthma nurse run the clinic together. The main advantage of such clinics is that they usually provide more time to talk. There are many things to learn about asthma, and these can't be dealt with easily in a busy surgery with 5- or 10-minute appointment times.

The clinic setting allows more time to deal with questions or concerns, particularly for people whose asthma has only recently been diagnosed. This book answers many of the questions that crop up repeatedly, but it is also helpful to talk to someone experienced in dealing with asthma.

A major problem in asthma care results from the difficulties in arranging regular follow-up and monitoring of people with asthma. These may occur because:

- the GP doesn't seem to have the time
- the GP doesn't think follow-up is needed
- the GP doesn't offer follow-up appointments
- the person with asthma doesn't take up the offer of an appointment
- the person with asthma feels well and fails to keep the appointment.

An asthma clinic offers some solutions to these problems. It is often more convenient and less crowded than a hospital clinic.

Community pharmacists are also beginning to be involved in sharing asthma care with the doctor and nurse in some areas, which is an exciting development. The practice nurse can check that the people on the practice *asthma register* are offered regular appointments to be seen, arrange flu vaccinations once a year, and make contact with people who do not attend.

Can my husband be referred for tests to see what's causing his asthma?

Your question makes us think you would also like to know more about his asthma. If your husband is happy for you to go with him to his asthma clinic, it can help you to become more involved with his treatment. You don't say if your husband is already under the care of the nurse or doctor at your practice. If he is, he needs to talk to them about any concerns he may have about his asthma. It is possible that some tests can be carried out at the practice.

The actual cause of asthma is not fully understood but there are trigger factors (see Chapter 2) that can set it off or make it worse. Triggers that start asthma off in the first place are called *allergens*. For example, someone exposed to latex powder may develop antibodies to it: he or she is now sensitised (but not yet allergic) to latex powder. If a sensitised person then has symptoms when exposed to the latex – or other allergenic substances (e.g. perfumes, pollens, food) – they are now allergic. Substances or situations that make asthma worse are also called *triggers*; for example, exercise, laughter, dust, fumes, pollens, open gas fires). Some of these triggers are known to the individual or the family and should be avoided where possible. Unfortunately, many people have multiple triggers and it is impossible to avoid them all.

If it seems likely, from talking to the doctor or asthma nurse, that your husband might be allergic to something, allergy tests can be done to confirm this. The most common type is called a *skin-prick test*, in which various substances, or allergens, are pricked into the skin. If the skin reacts and swells up, the person is probably allergic to that substance.

In most cases it is possible for the doctor to identify the trigger from talking to the person (taking a medical history), and allergy tests often just confirm a fact already known to the individual. However, these investigations may help to identify new trigger factors.

Special tests can measure the amount of *antibodies* (substances produced by the body's immune system) to certain allergens in the blood. If someone has an allergy that is important in causing symptoms, the levels of antibodies in the blood are very high.

Some occupations and environments are known to be linked with asthma and they can and do actually cause asthma. If your husband already has asthma, some working environments can make his asthma worse. The most common jobs associated with *occupational asthma* are:

- animal handlers
- bakers and pastry workers
- chemical workers
- food-processing workers
- nurses
- paint sprayers
- timber workers
- welders.

If your husband finds that his asthma is better when he is away from work or on holiday, it is possible that his job is making his asthma worse. He should talk to his nurse or doctor about this and, if an occupational trigger is suspected, he must be referred to a chest doctor specialising in occupational health as soon as possible.

What is the role of a practice nurse in preventing and treating asthma?

This depends a great deal on the practice and the individual nurse concerned. Many general practices now devote much more time to looking after people with asthma, and the practice nurse usually plays a major role.

Often there is a system of shared care between the doctor and the nurse but the nurse's role will depend on her or his knowledge of asthma and training in asthma management. So a practice nurse's involvement may range from a fairly minimal role – perhaps checking inhaler technique and understanding function tests – to a much higher level as is the case with an asthma specialist nurse, who has much more responsibility. In many practices, the role of the asthma nurse includes:

- obtaining a full asthma history
- recording and interpreting readings of peak expiratory flow/ understanding *spirometry*
- confirming, with the doctor, the diagnosis of asthma
- developing an appropriate asthma treatment and action plan in partnership with the individual and the doctor
- demonstrating, teaching and checking inhaler technique
- providing asthma education and counselling to enable people to manage their condition
- setting up a well-organised system for regular review of asthma symptoms, lung function tests, asthma medicines and inhaler devices
- being readily available to give advice, especially with worsening asthma
- treating acute asthma attacks according to current asthma guidelines.

Nurses should not take on this higher level of responsibility without receiving specialised training. Many practice nurses do have specific asthma training and have developed a high level of expertise. Their aim is to help people maintain optimum control of their asthma, and to minimise its effect on their lives. Some asthma nurses are also able to prescribe asthma medicines, after additional specialist training. You should feel able to ask about your nurse's training and expertise.

It is important that at least one doctor in the practice is also particularly interested in and knowledgeable about asthma. People with asthma will receive the most effective care if there is teamwork and good cooperation between the doctor, the asthma nurse, the pharmacist and the hospital.

How will I recognise if the asthma treatment is not working, and if more or a different treatment is needed?

The three most important clues that you need extra treatment are:

- if you are needing more than usual relief medication

- if you have worsening peak flow readings

- if you are having more symptoms than usual.

Anyone who needs to take reliever medication such as salbutamol (e.g. Ventolin or Airomir, albuterol) or terbutaline (Bricanyl) more than twice a week should be prescribed regular *preventer* asthma medicine, even if the asthma is usually mild and the medication is used only when symptoms occur. An increased need for salbutamol or terbutaline warns you that your asthma is out of control and that extra medicine is necessary.

- If you are already using one of the preventer inhaler medicines, and you find that you need to use your reliever inhaler more than twice a week, either your dose of preventer inhaler needs to be increased or other asthma treatment should be added.

- If your reliever inhaler medicine gives relief for less than 4 hours, this is a sign that your asthma is out of control. If your reliever medicine does not work quickly, or its effects last for less than 4 hours, your asthma is uncontrolled and medical help is needed. Take extra reliever while waiting for help and advice.

The fact that you need extra doses of the reliever medicines can provide useful information for your doctor or asthma nurse. This information, as well as your asthma symptoms and peak flow readings, will help your doctor to decide whether you need a change of treatment such as the addition of a preventer medicine.

Peak flow readings can also help you tell if your asthma treatment is not working. If the readings vary widely, this is another sign that your asthma is out of control.

Therefore, recognising that you need to use more reliever inhalers, or that they are not giving the usual relief as well as changes in your peak flow readings, will help you to recognise when to:

- adjust your own medication

- call for help.

How can I prevent an asthma attack?

Most asthma attacks can be prevented, but some cannot. Three things are key to preventing attacks:

- avoid your known trigger factors if at all possible

- recognise your early-warning signs

- take urgent action when they happen.

Take extra reliever treatment as soon as possible and call for medical help as soon as you notice that the treatment does not work. Most severe attacks can be prevented by these actions. You should discuss your own circumstances and actions with your doctor or asthma nurse, and agree a personal asthma action plan together.

Important signs of uncontrolled asthma are:

- increased symptoms

- lowered *peak expiratory flow* readings (PEFs)

- an increase in the gap between the morning and evening readings (*morning dipping*)

- PEF readings dropping steadily.

The charts in Figures 5.4, 5.5, 5.6 and 5.7 later in this chapter give examples of these changes.

PEAK EXPIRATORY FLOW MONITORING

Why do I need to use a peak flow meter?

Because it gives you a lot of information about your asthma! Measuring the peak flow can help to show you when an attack is on the way, how bad the attack is and also when your peak flow readings are better.

The peak flow meter in Figure 5.1 gives a reading (peak expiratory flow, or PEF) that tells you how open or tight your airways are. The more widely open the airways, the faster air can be blown out of the lungs when you breathe out forcefully, and the higher the PEF reading. Normal PEF readings vary for adult men and women

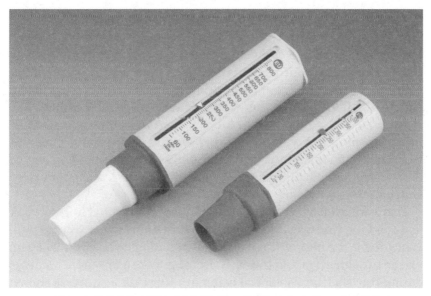

Figure 5.1 Mini-Wright Peak Flow Meters (adult and child)

depending on their age, sex, ethnicity and height. However, there is a very wide range of 'normal' PEF values, and most doctors and nurses will use the person's 'best-ever' peak flow reading as the normal one. *It is important for you to know your own best-ever peak flow reading, so that you can tell when it is low.* During episodes of uncontrolled asthma – whether they are attacks or exacerbations (worsenings) – the airways become narrowed and the PEF falls.

The PEF will often show a drop in readings a few days before symptoms develop. This helps you to decide when to increase your asthma medicines to prevent an attack or episode of uncontrolled asthma. The PEF can also help in confirming that your asthma control is good. If your PEF readings are normal for you, and there is very little change from day to day, your asthma is well controlled.

Another advantage of having your own peak flow meter is that you can check your progress when recovering from an asthma attack. The peak flow readings can help you tell when you are better. Once the readings are back to normal, it is safe to stop taking emergency medication (steroids and higher doses of inhaled medicines).

I have a peak flow meter, but what is a normal reading?

' Normal' readings are usually shown in a chart inside the box containing your peak flow meter. These readings depend on your age, sex, height, weight and ethnic group, but there is a problem with using them because there is a very wide range of 'normal'.

We prefer to use the *best* value achieved by someone instead of using 'normal' PEF values. In other words, each person finds out what their own *tailor-made normal* readings are. This reading can be used to tell if the asthma is well controlled or not when compared with day-to-day readings.

There are a few ways to find out your best or personal normal peak flow reading. One way is to keep a peak flow chart when you are well. Write down the best of three peak flow readings when you wake up and do the same again in the early evening. Take a few more readings during the day if possible. You can mark these on a chart, as shown in Figure 5.2. This graph, in a person with well-controlled asthma,

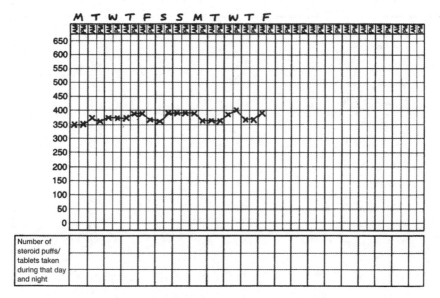

Figure 5.2 Finding your 'best ever' peak flow reading using a graph. This graph, in a person with well-controlled asthma, can be used to determine the 'best ever' peak expiratory flow (PEF). Here the readings average around 370, and this number could be used as the 'best ever' PEF.

can be used to determine the 'best ever' peak expiratory flow (PEF). In Figure 5.2 the readings average around 370, and this could be used as the 'best ever' PEF.

Alternatively, if you are not happy using graphs, the readings can be written down as we have shown in Figure 5.3.

Look at the readings and see what they are when you are at your best. Whilst it is easy to see the best readings in Figure 5.2, in Figure 5.3 the readings vary from 200 to 400 litres per minute (l/min) and it is difficult to say what that person's 'best readings' are. In this case it would be best to first get the asthma under control and then try to find out what the best readings are when well.

It may take some time to establish your best readings, but knowing your personal best peak flow is more accurate than using the normal

Day	Morning readings (best of 3)	Evening readings (best of 3)
Monday 25th	230	200
Tuesday 26th	300	350
Wednesday 27th	300	330
Thursday 28th	350	350
Friday 29th	330	270
Saturday 30th	320	300
Sunday 31st	350	320
Monday 1st	250	250
Tuesday 2nd	300	290
Wednesday 3rd	250	340
Thursday 4th	280	250

Figure 5.3 Finding your 'best ever' peak flow reading using a list of readings. Here the readings have been written down in a table.

readings provided in the packaging with the meter. The ideal time to find out your best reading is when you are well or possibly after taking a short course of steroid tablets for an attack. For example, look at Figure 5.4: the readings are normally about 300; they drop to 150 during the attack and then return to 350 after taking steroid tablets. This person's 'best PEF' is 350. If there are a few very high readings, while the majority are a bit lower, it is best to use the most common high reading as your best.

At what times of day should I record my peak expiratory flow?

The peak flow reading is usually at its lowest in the early hours of the morning and at its highest some time between mid-day and evening. If you record your PEF twice daily before any reliever treatment, this will give you a good picture of your asthma control. The best times are in the morning, soon after waking, and in the afternoon or early evening. If you cannot do afternoon readings, do

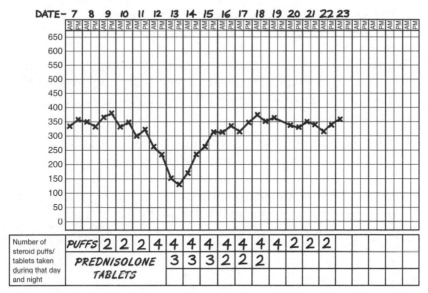

Figure 5.4 The readings are normally about 300; they then drop to 150 during the attack and then return to 350 after taking steroid (cortisone) tablets.

them during the early evening. Make a note of the best of three blows whenever you take your PEF. Morning readings alone are helpful, but it is really best to do afternoon or evening readings as well, because they will show how your asthma control changes during 24 hours.

How do I do a peak flow chart, and how do I know if my asthma is OK?

Your peak expiratory flow (PEF) readings can be written down in a simple number form such as in Figure 5.3 or in the form of a chart or graph as in Figures 5.2 and 5.4. When you take your PEF, do three of the best possible blows that you can and make a note of the highest of those three.

When asthma is well controlled, normal peak flow readings should stay roughly the same and be almost level. Compare Figure 5.2, which shows a nice level pattern, with the readings in Figure 5.5, which shows the very uneven lines of someone with uncontrolled asthma.

Figure 5.3 shows that the PEF readings are sometimes very low and at other times much higher. It is not difficult to see that this person's asthma is out of control. There are two key indicators of this poor control. Look at:

- The highest and the lowest readings. In Figure 5.3 the lowest reading is 200 and the highest is 400 – the highest reading is double the lowest. When asthma is well controlled, there should be very little difference between the day-to-day readings or between the morning and evening readings (less than 20%, and usually less than 10%).

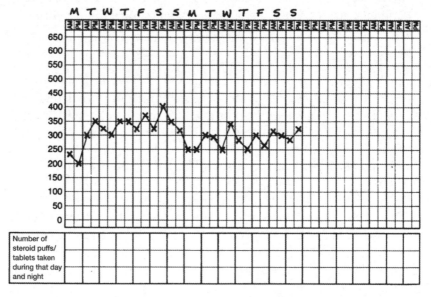

Figure 5.5 The readings for a child whose asthma is clearly out of control. They change from morning to evening and from day to day.

- The difference between the morning and the evening readings on the same days. Have a look at Figure 5.5, showing the readings for a child whose asthma is clearly out of control. The readings change from morning to evening and from day to day. In this chart, morning and evening values are almost the same at times and at other times very different. This gives an idea of the variation from morning to night, which is called the *diurnal variation*.

How useful can a peak flow meter be?

A peak flow meter is very useful because it gives a measurement of how tight your airways are. The readings can be used to see if your asthma is well controlled or uncontrolled. They can also show you how bad your asthma is sometimes, and even give a danger warning signal. Peak flow readings can also help you to use a personal asthma action plan in changing medication. We give you some examples of these uses in the next few answers.

When your asthma is well controlled, your twice-daily readings should be almost the same every time they are taken, although the evening reading is usually very slightly higher. The readings should not vary by more than about 20%. An example of a peak flow chart showing good asthma control can be seen in Figure 5.2. As discussed in the previous answer, the main indicator that your asthma is uncontrolled is when the readings change a lot from day to day. Figures 5.5, 5.6 and 5.7 show PEF readings of poorly controlled asthma.

Peak flow readings can also help to warn of really dangerous situations. Two patterns of peak flow readings indicate danger and a need to see a doctor urgently. The first is shown in Figure 5.6, where the readings are 'dipping down' early in the morning. The early-morning dips in peak flow on this chart on the 8th, 11th, 15th and 21st of the month were very serious warnings of uncontrolled asthma. This person needed additional treatment, and the doctor was consulted urgently.

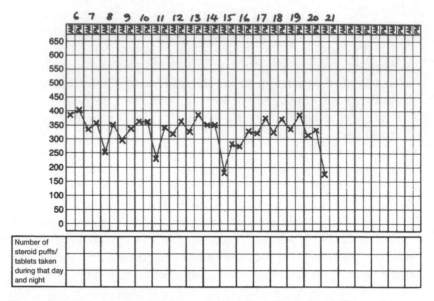

Figure 5.6 There are dangerous early-morning dips in peak flow – they are very serious warnings of poorly controlled asthma.

Figure 5.7 shows the second type of danger: the readings are dropping fast – a clear warning that an asthma attack may follow. Someone with a chart like this needs urgent medical help.

Another way that peak flow readings can help is in having a self-management plan. Figure 5.8 shows a 7-year-old child's peak flow chart. (Many children over the age of 5 are able to use a peak flow meter.) At the left side, where the chart starts, there are increased gaps between the morning and evening readings; this helped her mother to use the plan to start cortisone tablets, which have clearly helped to improve her asthma. The peak flow readings helped this child in two ways. The first was by showing her response to prednisolone (steroid) tablets. Second, the chart helped her mother to decide when it was safe to stop the steroid tablets – once the readings came back to the best levels.

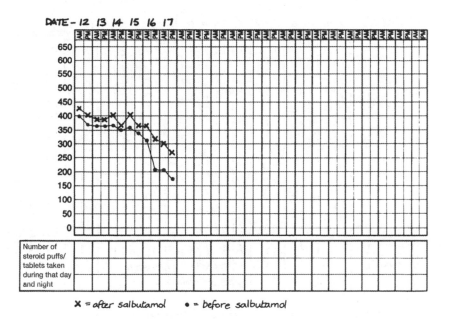

X = after salbutamol   • = before salbutamol

Figure 5.7 The readings are dropping fast – a danger warning. Someone with a chart like this needs urgent medical help.

My child is 3 years old, and on regular asthma treatment. When can he start to use a peak flow meter effectively?

Even though your son is only 3 years of age, he may be able to use a peak flow meter, but it is very unusual for children as young as this to be able to do so accurately. It may be better, for now, to monitor his asthma symptoms rather than peak flow readings. Of course, if he is able to get a few similar readings when he blows, he can use a meter. However, there is no value in peak flow readings if they are inaccurate and unreliable.

Very young children can be confused between breathing in to take their inhaler treatment and blowing out to record their PEF. If this happens, they may not take their treatment effectively. It is better to abandon the peak flow readings until they can easily separate the two

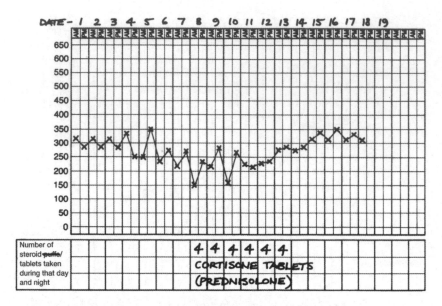

Figure 5.8 This 7-year-old child's peak flow chart shows increased gap between the morning and evening readings, and his response to prednisolone (steroid) tablets. The chart helps to decide when it is safe to stop the steroid tablets once the readings return to the best levels.

actions. Most children are unable to record a reading reliably until they are 5 or 6 years of age. Certainly by the age of 7 they should be able to use a peak flow meter.

Why do peak expiratory flow readings vary so much in the mornings, and why do people with asthma have a 'morning dip'?

In this sense, 'morning dip' is nothing to do with a trip to the local swimming pool! Asthma symptoms do tend to be worse during the early hours of the day, and the PEF is usually at its lowest at this time (see Figure 5.6).

There are many theories as to the cause of the morning dip, but no certainty. Possible explanations include posture when asleep, leakage of acid from the gullet into the airways, low body steroid levels during the night, and even low levels of body growth hormone during the night. Many careful research studies have investigated this problem but have not yet provided definite answers. (The readings are usually highest sometime between mid-day and the early evening.)

In practical terms, the size of the morning dip gives a good idea of how poorly the asthma is controlled. Treatment aims to remove, or at least minimise, the morning dip. People whose asthma is well controlled see little or no dip in the morning PEF reading.

This is why it is best to make at least two measurements of PEF during each day to assess the amount of morning dip, because it will vary from person to person.

WRITTEN PERSONAL ACTION PLANS FOR ASTHMA

What is a personal asthma action plan?

Personal asthma action plans are also known as 'self-management plans' and have been used increasingly in the past few years. The title is rather grand, but an action plan is simply an agreement between you and your doctor or nurse about the steps you can take to deal with your symptoms before calling for medical help. In this way, you become much more involved in the day-to-day control of your condition, and can respond to changing needs for treatment.

These sorts of agreements have existed for years but recently the emphasis has changed in two important ways:

- First, it is much more likely that plans will be written down. A range of cards, charts and booklets has been developed to enable the plan to be written down clearly.

- Second, in most cases (except for young children), PEF readings will form an important part of the plan so that, at certain peak flow levels, changes in treatment can be implemented. These levels will vary from person to person, depending on a number of factors. For example, your plan might say that you should start a course of prednisolone tablets if your PEF reading drops below 250, when it is normally between 480 and 520. In this case, you would start this course of treatment without needing to see your doctor or asthma nurse first.

Please note that the figures and treatments we give here are only examples, and you should not use them to manage your own asthma. Discuss the content of your plan with your own doctor or asthma nurse.

Some plans are quite complex, with a number of steps that may be taken, depending on changes in symptoms and PEF readings. Others are much more simple – saying, for example, 'If your PEF reading falls below 50% of your best reading, take 2–10 puffs of your reliever inhaler, and see a doctor or nurse urgently.'

In Figure 5.8, the child's usual peak flow was around 300 litres per minute (l/min). When the reading dropped to 150 l/min, her mother started her on cortisone tablets, which was recommended in her personal asthma action plan.

Research has found that asthma action plans work better if they:

- are written down

- use the personal best readings rather than general 'normal' readings

- have recommendations for the use of both inhaled and oral steroids.

Why should I work out the percentages on my action (self-management) plans?

Calculating a percentage target for PEF is a useful way to guard against uncontrolled asthma. The idea is to discover the best peak flow that you can achieve, and then use this as a 'benchmark' or standard against which action levels can be calculated. Where you place the dividing lines depends on your particular asthma, and that's why we call these plans 'personal asthma action plans'.

If you take PEF readings regularly, you will soon establish what your best reading is when you are well and completely free of symptoms. Various action levels for increasing treatment are calculated, depending on the system your doctor or nurse follows.

Figure 5.9 has an example of action levels. Assuming that well-controlled asthma is where the peak flow varies by less than 20%, the first action level could be set at 80% of your best reading. So if your best reading is 500 litres per minute (l/min), your first action level is set at 400 l/min (i.e. 80% of 500). Therefore, if your peak flow drops below 400 l/min, you need to take action. The action is what you agree with your doctor or nurse; it may be to increase your medication, or even to consult your doctor to check your medication.

Further lines can be set at 50% and 30% of your best reading. At 50% (200 l/min in this case) your agreed action plan may indicate that you start taking cortisone (prednisolone) tablets and consult your doctor or nurse. Figure 5.4 shows how someone added cortisone

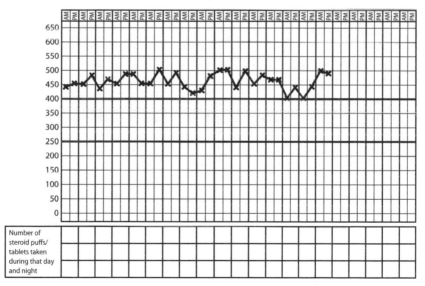

Figure 5.9 A peak flow chart with action levels drawn at 80% (400 l/min) and 50% (250 l/min) in a man whose best reading is about 500 l/min.

tablets when their readings dropped and this helped to prevent an asthma attack. If you agree a 30% level with your doctor – in this example, 130 l/min – you may be advised to call for emergency medical help or go directly to hospital if your peak flow drops to this level.

Figure 5.9 has some action lines showing how that person could see that their asthma was going out of control and also when to add additional medication or call for help. Personal asthma action plans are not meant to be too strict, and in this case the person might have added the cortisone tablets when the readings started dipping towards the 50% line rather than waiting till they reached that level. So the lines are meant as a guide to help a person with asthma judge when to take more medication, when to see their doctor and when to call for emergency assistance.

ALTERING AND CHANGING TREATMENT

Am I allowed to alter my treatment myself, or should my doctor always do this?

Doctors and nurses who have an interest in asthma aim to help their patients become expert in managing their own asthma. Thus, a major role for the health professional is to enable people to take care of their asthma themselves, while consulting with them regularly to reinforce this independence. This means that a clear personal action plan must be agreed. This will usually include the following information:

- Extra asthma medication to be taken if you are likely to be exposed to known asthma triggers.

- Common symptoms of asthma that indicate the need for an increase in asthma medicines.

- Continuing at the increased dose for a while until recovery takes place. The length of time will vary from one individual to another and between different episodes of asthma. (There are no fixed rules, only guidelines. In these circumstances the use of peak flow readings and charts may be very helpful.)

- Guidelines on when urgent medical help should be sought if the increased asthma medicine fails to improve the symptoms.

This type of personal asthma action plan is called 'guided self-management'. It means that you can alter your treatment if your symptoms or PEF readings change, according to your agreed plan. There is a section on asthma action plans (also known as self-management plans) earlier in this chapter.

Consult your doctor or asthma nurse if problems arise and your self-treatment is not working.

How long do I need to take my medicine for?

This depends on your age and other factors. Asthma is generally a lifelong condition. People do not outgrow their asthmatic tendency, although the disease often goes quiet for a while, perhaps for many years. This is called the *remission* phase of asthma. Unfortunately, however, it will sometimes flare up again in later life after exposure to an obvious trigger; more often it flares up for no apparent reason.

Asthma can be unpredictable and, because of this, you may be helped best by taking continuous treatment aimed at preventing the inflammation process in your airways. This treatment may be needed for a long time – possibly even years – after your symptoms have 'gone quiet'. If your asthma has gone into a truly prolonged remission, your treatment could be reduced or even stopped.

Ideally you should use peak flow readings for guidance when reducing or stopping treatment. Resume the treatment if your symptoms come back.

In adults, asthma treatment is usually for life. However, some adults get only short episodes of asthma; once these have cleared up completely, with little variation of the PEF, it is worth reducing or stopping the treatment. The use of a peak flow chart in this situation can be very helpful in deciding whether treatment should be resumed.

> *Can we decrease our son's asthma medicines? He has just had his 7th birthday, and has been well for 2 months.*

P ossibly, but discuss it with your doctor or asthma nurse because the dosage of medicine may be just right to control your son's symptoms. Two months without problems is very encouraging, but it may be a little soon to adjust his treatment; between 3 and 6 months is preferable.

For children, most doctors would advise treatment for at least 6 months or at least while symptoms remain. If your son is able to use a peak flow meter, daily peak flow readings will make sure that all is well. Treatment might be stopped, and restarted only if the readings continue to vary by more than 20%. Some children may not have any further trouble from their asthma, but the family should be aware that it could flare up suddenly, even after a number of symptom-free years. This is why it is so important to have a written personal action plan and get enough asthma medicine when you go on holiday, just in case.

In our view, once children have started asthma treatment, they should continue taking medication for at least a few months after symptoms have resolved. The main factor is the initial severity of the asthma. If, after a period of treatment, the asthma is very mild and there are few symptoms or attacks, therapy might be stopped. In older children, this may be done with the help of a peak flow chart, which provides early warning of deteriorating asthma.

If it is decided to reduce or stop the treatment, it may be better to wait until after the coughs and colds season because they are the main asthma triggers in children. However, bear in mind that the end of that season also heralds the hay fever season, if this sort of allergy is a problem for him.

We believe that peak flow meter readings are very helpful. A chart will show whether it is safe to decrease your son's asthma medicines.

A level peak flow chart such as the one in Figure 5.2, in which the graph is almost a straight line, would indicate that the asthma is well controlled. In this case you could try reducing his medicine, and then monitor the peak flow readings. If the readings stay level, and there are no symptoms, it is safe to continue on the lower dose. However, if the readings begin to vary, the control of asthma is being lost, and the previous dose should be taken again.

As a general rule, peak flow readings should not go up or down by more than 20%. The formula to calculate this change (variation) is shown in Chapter 3 (at the bottom of page 33).

If the change is greater than 20%, the variation is too high and his asthma is out of control. For example, if his highest reading during the week is 400 and the lowest is 300, the peak flow variation is 25%, which indicates that the asthma is quite badly out of control.

As long as the peak flow readings do not go up or down by more than 20%, it is safe to stay on the lower dose. In a few more months it may be possible to make another reduction in the treatment.

Is it better for me to put up with my asthma, and not take any asthma medicines?

No, and if putting up with asthma means that you are having symptoms, the answer is definitely no. The presence of asthma symptoms means the presence of inflammation of the airways, and treatment will help relieve this.

Asthma inflammation is an ongoing process, which can damage the lungs. It also makes the asthma more liable to flare up and result in an attack. We feel that people whose asthma is causing them regular symptoms should be taking regular anti-asthma medicines that reduce the underlying inflammation.

Such *preventer* medicines include those described in Chapter 4: beclometasone (e.g. Becotide), budesonide (e.g. Pulmicort), fluticasone (Flixotide), mometasone (Asmanex), ciclesonide (Alvesco).

Nedocromil sodium (Tilade) and sodium cromoglicate (Intal) are used less often nowadays in the UK and Europe, because inhaled steroids usually work better. However, they may be appropriate for some people.

Another preventer drug comes in the form of a tablet or a powder that can be sprinkled on food. This group of preventer drugs are called *leukotriene receptor antagonist* (or LTRA) drugs. They are described in Chapter 4.

When can I stop my steroid tablets after an attack?

U sually they are taken for between 5 and 10 days but this varies, so it is essential to see your doctor within a few days of being treated for an attack. The best way to decide this is with the help of a peak flow meter and a daily peak flow chart. Most health professionals now accept that people with asthma can follow a personal action plan for self-management once one has been agreed between those involved. (There is a section on personal asthma action plans earlier in this chapter, and information on managing emergencies is given in Chapter 8.)

The basic guidelines for a personal action plan follow.

- The usual peak expiratory flow reading is taken as the normal or best reading. If, as is preferable, you have your own meter, you will usually have a good idea of your best or normal readings.

- If your morning and evening readings show a wide difference (more than 20%), you should follow your agreed action plan. This will probably include increasing your preventer medication (inhaled steroid) by four or five times and, of course, taking more reliever medication as needed, until your readings no longer vary by so much from morning to evening (or from day to day).

- When the PEF drops below 40%–60% of your best reading (as advised in your asthma action plan), you will normally be offered a course of steroid tablets. The dose is usually 30–60 mg/day in adults (20 mg/day for children aged 2–5 years; 30–40 mg/day for children over 5 years).

- The tablets are continued at the daily dose until the peak flow reaches your best or normal value. It is important to keep taking these tablets until a good response has been achieved – the time this takes is different for everyone. A peak flow chart is very helpful in deciding when it is safe to stop taking these tablets – usually when the readings have got back to the 'best ever' and stayed the same for a few days. (In young children, 3 days' treatment is often sufficient to gain control of asthma symptoms.)

- See your asthma nurse or doctor frequently after an attack until you are better, and you will soon learn how to deal with any future attacks.

Figure 5.4 shows where someone took cortisone (steroid) tablets until he was better and his peak flow readings returned to his usual best levels. With the help of the chart, he was also able to tell when his peak flows were almost back to the usual best readings and it was safe to stop the tablets.

How can I recognise that my treatment is working?

You can tell that your treatment is working when your symptoms improve and your peak flow chart has returned towards normal. Another way you can tell is when you find that you do not need to use more than two puffs a week of your rescue (*reliever*) mediation.

The use of a daily peak flow chart is particularly helpful when new treatment has been started or when the dose of existing treatment is increased. Signs of improvement on the chart are:

- your readings are fairly constant, without variation from morning to evening, and from day to day

- your readings are improving towards your normal or 'best' values.

Personal action plan – things you might wish to discuss with your doctor or asthma nurse

Once you have read through this chapter, there may be a number of things you might wish to discuss with your doctor or asthma nurse. These may include:

- asking for a prescription for a peak flow meter and learning how to keep a peak flow chart

- finding out what triggers your asthma and how to prevent exposure to these triggers

- finding out how often you should consult the doctor or nurse for asthma check-ups

- checking that you are on the right asthma medicines and whether the dose needs to be adjusted

- agreeing a personal asthma action plan for yourself (or your child), and ensuring you have the right asthma medicines

- knowing what to do if you have a severe asthma attack

- finding out how your doctor's practice works and how you:
  - arrange a routine check-up
  - obtain a repeat prescription
  - get help in an emergency.

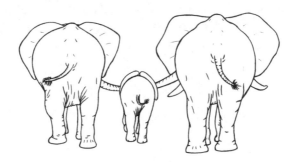

6 | Living with asthma

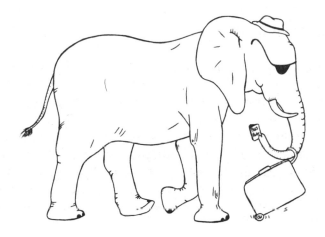

In this chapter you will learn about:

- how to manage your asthma

- why asthma does not need to rule your life

- asthma and work

- asthma and food allergy

- physical fitness and asthma

- holidays.

While it is important to try to avoid things that make your asthma worse, asthma does not have to rule your life. This chapter deals with some of the very practical questions that worry people with asthma. There are several sections in this chapter, dealing with different aspects of the environment in which we live.

Holidays should be a time for you to enjoy yourself, rather than thinking about your asthma. Good planning can prevent problems from occurring because of acute asthma attacks in faraway places.

EVERYDAY LIFE

Why is my asthma at its worst when I carry heavy shopping?

Carrying shopping is a strenuous activity, and any strenuous exercise or activity may trigger asthma symptoms.

If exercise makes your asthma worse only on occasions such as this, you could prevent it by taking an extra dose of *reliever* medication just before doing something physical. However, this symptom may be a warning sign that your asthma is not well controlled. If so, you may need to start *preventer* treatment or to use more if you are already taking it.

If you have to take your reliever medicine more than twice a week for asthma symptoms, you probably need more preventer medicine treatment. Talk to your doctor or nurse about this.

There are sections on treatment in Chapter 4 and on action plans for self-management in Chapter 5.

Why is asthma often bad at night?

This is very common, and indeed symptoms at night are a good indicator that your asthma is not well controlled. You should not have any night-time symptoms. They result in disrupted sleep, so you probably feel tired in the morning. A bad asthma attack at night can also be very frightening.

We don't know for sure why night-time symptoms occur, but there are several theories. The most common possible explanation is related to normal body physiology in that we produce lower levels of certain body hormones at night (particularly cortisone and growth hormone).

Perhaps the most important likely explanation is that a change takes place in the body's natural rhythms during the night. These are known as *circadian rhythms*. Everyone (whether or not they have asthma) has an individual lung function pattern during a 24-hour period. Peak flow readings are commonly lower first thing in the morning whilst others might be high during the morning. On average, though, the best (highest) readings are between mid-day and 14:00.

In poorly controlled asthma, the early-morning readings are usually much lower, and breathing can worsen dramatically at this time. Remember that, if your asthma wakes you up, it is out of control! The low readings of early morning match the low point for hormones that are produced by the body, and the two are probably connected. We still have much to learn about asthma at night but one thing we can say for sure is that good day-time control leads to improvements in night-time asthma.

There are a few other possible explanations for asthma problems at night but research at present does not substantiate them. They include:

- posture, as we tend to lie flat at night
- dust and house dust mites in the bedding, triggering asthma symptoms
- increased acid production by the stomach
- changes in air and body temperature.

I sometimes wheeze when I go near a dog, or when it is very dusty. Is this an allergy or asthma?

It is probably both – asthma symptoms triggered by your allergies. Dogs and dust are both important and common triggers of asthma symptoms. The allergic reaction to the dog or dust may make you wheeze and cause an asthma attack if it is not treated promptly.

As well as triggering asthma, there may be other signs of allergy, especially itching skin, runny nose and sneezing, and itchy eyes.

Why do I wheeze when I go into a warm house from the cold outside?

Changes of temperature are responsible for making you wheeze, particularly when your airways are irritable and sensitive. A sharp change in temperature may set off an asthma attack. It may be that your symptoms begin outside in the cold but become worse when you get indoors.

Cold air is a well-known trigger of asthma symptoms, and going from a warm house to the open air in the winter frequently makes people cough and wheeze.

Other allergens such as dusts, moulds or animal hairs may also trigger your symptoms as you move indoors.

At the beginning of the winter months when the central heating is switched on, my nasal passages feel very tickly. What can I do about it?

Before we explain what you can do to help to alleviate this problem, let us explain why it might happen. There are two likely explanations for these symptoms: one is allergy to the house dust mite, and the other is the onset of cold winter weather. The second is the condition called *rhinitis*. Many people with asthma also suffer from rhinitis.

In *allergic rhinitis* the lining of the nasal passages reacts to trigger factors (*allergens*), in just the same way that the lining of the airways does in asthma. The reaction may be a tickly sensation, a feeling of being 'blocked up' or even a runny nose with frequent sneezing. There are many possible allergens, but in your case house dust mite allergy is the most likely cause. Another well-known allergen is grass pollens, which cause *hay fever*.

Although the house dust mite causes problems throughout the year, the numbers are at their highest during the early winter months. Switching on the central heating gives a boost to their numbers by raising the temperature. Warm, centrally heated houses with fitted carpets and curtains provide an almost-perfect environment for house dust mite numbers to multiply! So it might be worth looking at alternative flooring options in some parts of the house. We can't really suggest that you turn off your central heating, as that would not be practical!

Ironically, cold weather is another trigger factor for rhinitis. This is not a true allergy, but is usually called *vasomotor rhinitis*. Cold air causes a reaction in the lining of the nose, with results similar to those of allergy.

If your rhinitis is very troublesome, we suggest that you talk to your doctor, nurse or pharmacist about it. There are several highly effective treatments, and most of them are available without a prescription ('over the counter').

What about keeping pets? I have asthma and my children want a cat – do I go ahead and get them one?

If you have asthma and you are sensitive to certain animals, your asthma may be worse if they live in your home. Having pets to which you are allergic is not a good idea. However, it isn't really possible to tell if you would be affected.

Perhaps your children could visit friends or neighbours who have animals. Some animal owners might be glad of help with looking after them, such as taking a dog for walks. Your children could enjoy the company of animals without the risk of making your asthma worse.

SMOKING

I have heard that girls and women suffer more from asthma than men if they smoke – is this true?

There is some research evidence that children of women who smoke in pregnancy are more at risk of developing asthma. We are not aware of any research that has confirmed that women or girls suffer more than men from their asthma.

Before puberty, asthma is more common in boys than in girls. After puberty, more women suffer from asthma, and there are many possible reasons for this; many young women smoke and that may be why some people associate the two.

I have heard that smoking doesn't affect asthma – is that true?

No, there is very strong evidence that asthma is made worse by either smoking yourself or being exposed to cigarette (or any tobacco) smoke. Asthma treatments do not work as well in people who smoke (or who are exposed to smoke); the dose of preventer needs to be increased. This applies particularly to children, who may have to endure smoky atmospheres through no fault of their own. In fact, there is a current campaign in the UK to try to stop people from smoking in their cars for this very reason.

Perhaps even more worrying is the evidence that smoking among pregnant women and mothers is causing their children to develop asthma symptoms.

How can I stop my husband from smoking in front of the children?

Parents who smoke are putting their children's health at risk, in both the short and the long term. People are often simply unaware of the risks posed by passive smoking – for example, the very high exposure of people travelling in cars with someone who is smoking. Perhaps if you can convince your husband of these facts he might be prepared to smoke away from areas of direct contact with your children.

There is increasing evidence for the harmful effects of cigarette/ tobacco smoke on children's asthma. We know that:

- infants exposed to passive cigarette smoke suffer from more wheezing illness during the first year of life than infants who are not exposed thus

- lung growth and lung function in children whose parents smoke are not as good as in those whose parents do not smoke

- cigarette smoke is a trigger factor for asthma attacks.

The problem is particularly bad for children with asthma whose parent(s) or relatives smoke in the home. Research suggests that children whose mothers smoke suffer most, and that this is far worse for children who are at home all day rather than away at school or nursery. The main risk factor seems to be the length of time the child spends with a smoker.

We are sure you will be aware that the issue of smoking can sometimes be a cause of friction in the family! If your husband is willing to stop smoking, encourage him to seek professional help.

SEX, PERIODS, PREGNANCY AND THE MENOPAUSE

Sex

Asthma seems to interfere with my sex life – why is this?

Although asthma is a common condition, it is not a frequent cause of sexual difficulties. However, poorly controlled asthma can affect your life in many ways, including your sexual relations. If asthma symptoms do occur during sex, they can cause problems. Symptoms can be brought on by:

- exertion; this reaction can prevented by using a reliever medicine (such as salbutamol or terbutaline) before intercourse

- movement in bed, which can sometimes cause large amounts of allergens to be released from the bedclothes, triggering wheezing

- allergy to a partner's semen (sperm), although this is very rare.

Allergy to latex condoms is also rare but can cause a generalised allergic reaction, which may include asthma. This can happen suddenly, with catastrophic results. It is called an *anaphylactic attack*, which could be life threatening. It can happen up to 6 hours later (also called a *late [allergic] reaction*). Latex-free condoms are available but anyone allergic to latex should consult an allergy specialist.

As far as we are aware, asthma medicines do not affect sexual desire or responses.

Periods

Could my periods have any sort of connection with my asthma symptoms?

Quite possibly, as it is likely that the menstrual cycle has an effect on asthma in many women. Research has found that, in some women, asthma gets worse during the week before a period (menstruation). This link between getting asthma symptoms before periods seems to be more of a problem in some women with severe or poorly controlled asthma. We know that such women can have severe asthma attacks around the time of menstruation.

Research has found a fall in peak expiratory flow (PEF) and an increase in symptoms at the time of menstruation in as many as one in three women with asthma. Remembering to take your *preventer* medicines regularly will help to keep your asthma under control.

If this situation is the case with you, you would benefit by monitoring your peak flow recordings and/or your asthma symptoms either regularly or in the week leading up to your period. Any changes in peak flow will alert you to take extra asthma medicines when needed.

A personal asthma action plan based on peak flow readings will be useful. This can also help to identify when to seek advice for poorly controlled asthma. (See the sections on peak expiratory flow in Chapters 3 and 5 and 'Written action plans for asthma' in Chapter 5.) Keep a peak flow diary of your readings for at least 3 months to see if there is a regular pattern of a consistent fall in PEF around or before your period. If so, that is strong evidence to support your suspicions and it would be sensible to increase your preventer treatment during the week before falls in peak flow are expected. If this does not help, you should see your asthma nurse or doctor.

Many women take pain killers and anti-inflammatory tablets for period pain, and this is another possible cause of poor control of your asthma during periods. Commonly used are aspirin and similar *anti-inflammatory drugs* such as ibuprofen (Nurofen) and mefenamic acid (Ponstan). They are all members of a large group of medicines known as non-steroidal anti-inflammatory drugs (*NSAIDs*) and they can cause symptoms of asthma, particularly in people who are allergic to or intolerant of aspirin. These pain-relief medicines are best avoided if you have asthma.

If you need to take regular medicines for period pains, check with your doctor, asthma nurse or pharmacist as to what may be suitable for you.

Pregnancy

What effect does being pregnant tend to have on my asthma?

Pregnancy has a variable effect on asthma. Research has found that, for some women, their asthma actually improves during pregnancy. During pregnancy, you have high levels of oestrogen in your blood, and for some women this may make asthma worse. Around 40% of women require more treatment to control their asthma during pregnancy, around 40% keep to the same treatment and around 20% actually need less.

Recent studies have found that the health of a newborn baby is unaffected by the mother having asthma. Any risk for the baby during pregnancy comes from uncontrolled asthma and severe acute attacks. It is important therefore to try to prevent this from happening. All pregnant women with asthma should have regular check-ups with the doctor or asthma nurse to make sure that their asthma is well controlled. This might mean increasing or changing medication.

Acute asthma attacks may cause a shortage of oxygen for both the mother and her growing baby, and this can be dangerous. It may result in smaller babies and even stillbirth after severe asthma attacks, although the latter is extremely rare. Inhaled corticosteroids, which are frequently used as reliever medications, are safe in pregnancy and are important in preventing asthma attacks.

I've just been told I am pregnant – can I still take my medication?

Yes, your inhaled medications can *and should be* taken as usual. Asthma attacks can be harmful for both mother and child, so it is very important to continue taking your asthma medication in pregnancy. In the first 3 months of pregnancy, the general rule is to avoid taking medicines by mouth (i.e. tablets or syrup) unless they are really necessary. Your doctor or nurse can advise you about this.

Asthma medicines that are taken by inhaler are safe during all stages of pregnancy. If you are already taking montelukast tablets for asthma, it is safe for you to continue taking them, but they should not be started during pregnancy, as there is not enough evidence to suggest that this is safe. If asthma is poorly controlled or you have an asthma attack, a short course of steroid tablets may be necessary – this is better than risking harming the baby through uncontrolled asthma.

It is very important for you to try to control your asthma during your pregnancy. If you have severe asthma attacks, the main risk to your baby is that he or she may be born underweight. In a very severe asthma attack, there is a tiny but real risk of infant death.

During pregnancy, regular peak flow monitoring and more frequent asthma check-ups will alert both you and your health professionals if your asthma is getting worse.

Will I get breathing difficulties in labour?

As long as your asthma is well controlled, your breathing should be no different from that of any other woman in labour. Towards the end of pregnancy, the womb (uterus) takes up a lot of extra space in the abdomen. This causes pressure, which pushes the diaphragm upwards and 'squeezes' the lungs. In late pregnancy and in labour, this results in breathing being slightly more difficult. If your asthma is bad, an extra strain will be placed on your breathing, and you may notice some difficulties. Talk to your health professional if you are worried about your asthma control in the later stages of your pregnancy.

You can help prevent breathing problems in labour by using the breathing exercises that you will be taught at antenatal classes, and by taking your asthma medication regularly.

The anxiety and excitement that occur when labour begins may result in your forgetting to take your asthma inhalers. You may even leave them at home in the rush to get to hospital! So it is a good idea to pack an extra inhaler in your maternity suitcase.

Will breastfeeding reduce the likelihood of my baby developing asthma, or its severity?

There is new research evidence that full breastfeeding during the first 4 months of life results in fewer children having asthma by the age of 4 years. Partial breastfeeding (mixed bottle and breast) does offer some protection but not as good as in the case of full breastfeeding.

Other research suggests that, of children who do develop asthma, those who were breastfed may get less severe asthma than those who were not breastfed. In addition, the evidence is quite strong that breastfeeding protects against the development of *atopic* eczema when there is a family history of the condition. Breastfeeding needs to continue for around 6 months to reduce the chances of the baby becoming allergic to cow's milk, and then developing *eczema*.

Over all, we believe that, with regard to asthma and allergies, it is much better if babies are breastfed if at all possible. This is particularly relevant if one or both parents are *atopic* or have asthma, and also if the child is exposed to tobacco smoke in the home.

Menopause

I am going through the menopause and my doctor has put me on hormone tablets because I am having lots of problems. Will it make my asthma worse?

Although lung function declines with increasing age, it is difficult to be certain what happens to asthma as women go through the menopause. There is some evidence that increased 'twitchiness' in the airways is associated with this treatment, which means an increased risk of asthma. We cannot be certain whether hormone replacement treatment (HRT) will have any effect on your asthma.

You don't say how severe or how well controlled your asthma is, but the better controlled your asthma is, the less likely you are to be troubled by the menopause or HRT.

Be sure to take your asthma treatment as discussed with your doctor or asthma nurse and have your asthma checked regularly.

I have read that steroid tablets cause brittle bones. Will my asthma inhalers cause the same problems?

Osteoporosis, or thinning of the bones, is a side-effect of long-term steroid tablets, but it also occurs as a result of hormonal changes that happen with increasing age: decreasing oestrogen levels in women and decreasing testosterone levels in men. An increased life span and decreasing hormone levels also increase the likelihood of bone (especially hip) fractures. A family history of osteoporosis is also a risk factor for that condition.

If you have difficult asthma and take steroid tablets regularly, you are likely to experience side-effects from them. Your inhalers are unlikely to have any effect on your bones if you are on less than 800 micrograms per day (µg/day) of inhaled steroid. If you are using higher doses or are having more than 4 weeks of treatment each year with oral steroid tablets, your bone density could be affected.

We recommend that you continue to take your asthma treatment, but also talk to your doctor or nurse about your concerns. It may be possible to reduce the dosage without loss of asthma control. They may also be able to arrange for you to have a special test to check for osteoporosis (called bone densitometry) and at the same time have a blood test to check your calcium and vitamin D levels.

I am on steroid inhalers for my asthma. Is there anything I can do to help protect my bones?

There are several ways to promote healthy bones:

- regular weight-bearing exercise (walking or running)

- stopping smoking if you are a smoker – there is help out there, as it is not easy

- keeping alcohol levels below recommended maximums (high alcohol intake increases the risk of having bone fractures)

- having a diet rich in calcium (lots of dairy products)

- get some sun on your skin from time to time; sunlight is needed to activate vitamin D which, together with calcium, helps to strengthen your bones.

If you are taking less than 800 micrograms per day (µg/day) of inhaled steroid, the risk of bone thinning from your asthma treatment is small. If your asthma is well controlled, talk to your asthma nurse or doctor to see if it is possible to reduce your treatment. It is often possible to reduce treatment without loss of asthma control.

WORK

How do different working conditions (e.g. air conditioning, smoky rooms) affect different people with asthma?

There are a number of working conditions that can have an effect on asthma. The type of work you do may be as important as your working conditions. Types of work that may affect asthma include working with:

- animals (e.g. farmers and vets)
- certain spices (e.g. mustard)
- dusts and fumes (e.g. open gas fires and gas cookers); see also Chapter 2.

Adequate ventilation in the workplace helps to reduce such problems.

As far as working conditions are concerned, anything that pollutes the air can make asthma worse. Air conditioning or heating may recirculate polluted air and increase problems rather than improve them. Fan-air central heating may spread virus infections (colds), which aggravate asthma.

What is occupational asthma?

There are two types of asthma that may occur as a result of your work. *Occupational asthma* is where asthma starts, for the first time, from repeated exposure to substances in the workplace (see below for a list of these). Most people with this type of asthma develop an allergy to substances being used in the workplace. The second type is where someone already has asthma but it becomes worse at work. This is called *work-aggravated asthma*.

If your asthma consistently improves at weekends or on days away from work, such as holidays, you may have occupational asthma and you should be referred to a specialist in this field. Your doctor or asthma nurse may ask you to keep a peak flow chart, every 4 hours, while you are waiting to see the specialist. You will need to do these peak flow readings when you are at work and at home. If your readings are better when away from work, this will support a diagnosis of occupational asthma.

Substances that may cause asthma in the workplace include:

- adhesives – in particular the isocyanates used in manufacturing polyurethane spray paints and surface lacquers – and epoxy resin hardening agents
- aldehydes (health professionals whose work involves sterilising instruments)
- animals and insects (laboratory workers, farmers, and veterinary workers)
- drugs: some drugs during manufacture – e.g. cimetidine and certain antibiotics
- dyes such as carmine
- flour, grain and coffee beans
- latex (health professionals in particular are at risk)
- metals – aluminium, cobalt, chrome, nickel, platinum salts and stainless steel
- proteolytic enzymes – in baking, meat tenderising and detergent manufacture.
- soldering flux (containing colophony or ammonium chloride)
- wood dusts, especially hardwoods (cabinet makers are more likely to develop occupational asthma than are general builders)

I have just started a new job in a bakery and my asthma has got worse. Why is this?

Asthma that gets worse at work, or *work-aggravated asthma*, is not uncommon. There are a number of occupations that can make asthma worse, and baking is one of these (see the list in the previous answer). You should ask your doctor or asthma nurse to refer you to a specialist in occupational medicine.

They might ask you to do a peak flow chart with readings every 4 hours (both at and away from work) for several weeks to try to see if you have occupational asthma. Doing this while waiting for the appointment can help save time when you see the specialist.

Will asthma affect my son's future employment?

With regard to employment, there is a small chance that a history of asthma may cause problems for young adults seeking work.

However, people with asthma are just as well qualified as those without, and should stand an equal chance of being employed. Ill-informed employers who believe that people with asthma are anxious (or 'nervous') types are discriminating against them unfairly.

Certain occupations or conditions in the workplace could have a bad effect on your son's asthma. Any job that involves close contact with dust, sprays, fumes or poor air quality should be avoided wherever possible, as should occupations where there is contact with any of the substances listed earlier in this section.

Ideally, your son's working environment should be free of cigarette smoke but we realise that it is not always possible to choose your workplace in countries where smoking isn't banned in public places. If he gets a job with a large organisation, he should be able to get help from the occupational health department or union representative in improving his working environment.

HOLIDAYS

Does travel cause any discomfort to people with asthma?

Asthma should not normally cause any particular problems during travel. One of the main risks is having an asthma attack and being caught off guard when away from home. This is much more important than any risk associated with the travel itself.

Any circumstances that cause a shortage of oxygen may increase respiratory symptoms and cause discomfort. A holiday where the altitude is above 6000–7000 feet may cause discomfort even for people who do not have asthma, but might be problematic for those with symptoms.

So enjoy your trip! It shouldn't cause problems but it is worth planning carefully.

Countries around the world have different arrangements for emergency medical care, and it is worth finding out about them and the need for medical insurance before you travel. For example, if you take a holiday in the UK it is possible to consult a National Health Service doctor in an emergency. This is the easiest and best way to get help unless you are unlucky enough to suffer a serious attack, when urgent transfer to an Accident and Emergency department is indicated. (See Chapter 8, 'Emergencies', for more about when to go straight to hospital.) If you do need to be referred to hospital for severe asthma, the doctor will know the arrangements for getting help quickly from the local specialist.

Make sure that you have adequate health insurance cover when travelling abroad. You will have to let the insurance company know about your asthma, and any other medical conditions you might have. If you don't mention all of your medical conditions, the policy might be invalid.

I am going on holiday, and don't want to take my inhalers with me. Is that all right?

No, it isn't! We will assume you are taking both preventer and reliever inhalers, so let's discuss them separately and we will give you reasons why you should take both of them on holiday with you. Put them in your carry-on luggage in case your other luggage gets lost.

It is really important that, if your doctor or asthma nurse has prescribed a *preventer* inhaler for you, you should use it on a regular basis, even if you are fit and well and have no current asthma symptoms. By not using your preventer inhaler regularly as advised, your asthma could get worse and go out of control and could ruin your holiday.

Your *reliever* inhaler is equally important and you should take it with you on holiday, keeping it with you at all times.

If you have an agreed personal asthma action plan (see Chapter 5), which includes advice on using short bursts of corticosteroid tablets for attacks, be sure to take an emergency pack with you whenever you go away. The emergency pack typically includes corticosteroid tablets, a peak flow meter, spare reliever and preventer inhalers, and, if needed, a letter from your doctor. Travelling to different parts of the country or the world may expose you to different asthma triggers, including changes in temperature. As a result, your asthma may deteriorate even if it is normally well controlled.

> *My inhaler is pressurised. The airline regulations say that I cannot carry it in my hand luggage, so what can I do? What if I need to use it during the flight?*

Although the regulations may state this, airlines do recognise that people with asthma need to take pressurised inhalers with them on their travels. It is preferable and safer for you to carry your treatment with you in your cabin hand luggage because you have the medication available if you need it. Moreover, if your luggage goes missing, you could lose your inhalers as well!

Some airlines, but not all, carry emergency asthma treatment on some of their flights. Check this with the airline or the travel company you will be using.

> *Can I get my usual inhaler in other countries?*

Some of the newer inhaler devices may be more difficult to obtain than the traditional *puffers* or aerosol inhalers, which are widely available throughout the world. Most asthma inhaler medicines are available in countries in western Europe, USA, Canada, Australia and New Zealand, with a doctor's prescription.

In an emergency, you could probably get a reliever inhaler over the counter (without a prescription) as you can in the UK. The formulation, strength and brand name of the medicine might vary slightly from country to country.

In the USA you may be able to obtain your usual asthma medicines, but not always. They may have different names and dose strengths, and you will need to have them prescribed by a doctor or nurse prescriber. In many countries of south-east Asia you can buy medicines from a pharmacy without a prescription.

Make sure that you know exactly what you want, and always check that the medicine is in date and has not been opened or tampered with. Also cross-check the *generic* names (not the brand or trade name) of your medication if buying it while travelling.

Medical information departments of the major pharmaceutical companies will be able to tell you which of their products are available in which countries and under what names. In addition, you could check some of this on the internet before you travel. Unless you are away for a long time, we suggest that you always take enough of your inhalers with you if you go abroad. Take at least one spare with you in case you lose the one you are using, and take any necessary emergency treatment with you, in case you have an acute asthma attack.

SPORT

Isn't it dangerous to use my inhaler before exercise?

No, it is not dangerous – quite the opposite is true. Using a *reliever* inhaler before exercise is quite safe, and will usually prevent asthma symptoms that are triggered during or after exercise.

However, if you need to use your reliever inhaler before exercise, your asthma is not controlled, and you should see your doctor because you will either need a preventer or a change of your preventer medicine.

Are there any sports that I should avoid taking part in?

You should be able to participate in most sports despite having asthma. However, scuba diving is one where the situation is not always very clear. Some doctors will advise you not to dive if you have asthma, because there is a risk of dying if you have an attack when underwater. In some countries you will not be allowed to dive if you have asthma. We advise anyone with asthma planning a diving holiday to find out the rules in the country they are travelling to, and also at the resort that they plan to visit.

Other sports that involve the use of pressurised air or oxygen, such as skydiving, might require caution, but you should take specialist advice on this. For the most part, assuming your asthma is well controlled, you should be able to participate in all other sporting activities.

If, like some people, you are affected by the chlorine used in many swimming pools, you should probably avoid swimming in them.

I play football (soccer). Is it all right to take two more puffs at half-time even though it's not 4 hours between doses?

It is perfectly safe to take two puffs of a *reliever* earlier than 4 hours from the last dose. However, needing to take your inhaler before and during exercise is an indication that your asthma is not well controlled and you should get a check-up from your doctor or nurse.

Regular preventive treatment may be necessary to control asthma symptoms effectively. However, if you need frequent reliever treatments, as for example on the playing field, some adjustment to your regular treatment is required.

Regular *peak expiratory flow* readings will help to determine whether your asthma is well controlled. If the readings vary by more than 20% a day, from morning to evening, it is wise to consult your doctor or asthma nurse.

If your asthma is well controlled, you will have more stamina on the field and your game should improve!

POLLUTION AND WEATHER

Are pollutants in the air causing asthma?

Surprisingly, the answer is 'Probably not'. The highest levels of asthma in the world are found in New Zealand, hardly a candidate for the world's most polluted country! Much research on the incidence of asthma around the world has found lower levels of asthma in more polluted cities. For example, the incidence of asthma was much lower in the former East German cities (that had very polluted atmospheres) than in old West Germany. Similarly, London in the 1950s had little asthma, but was a far more polluted city than it is now.

Nevertheless, there is something about urbanisation and the increasing incidence of asthma, and it cannot be good for anyone to breathe in air that is of poor quality. So the full answer is that air pollution does worsen asthma, but does not explain the increases in asthma cases that we have seen in the past 55 years.

Outdoors, there are three major sources of pollutants in the air that we breathe:

- fumes from exhausts of motor vehicles that use petrol (even unleaded) or diesel fuel

- smoke produced from burning coal, wood and gas (factories, industries and home coal fires are largely responsible for this form of pollution)

- ground-level *ozone*, which is formed by a reaction between the sun's rays and other forms of pollution such as car exhaust fumes; smoke from cigarettes/tobacco, factories and fires; paint and glue fumes; and fog.

Ozone is a gas, related to oxygen, that is found in small quantities in the air. This ground-level ozone is harmful to the lungs, and our pollution is producing more of it. It helps to form what is called *photochemical smog*. All of these conditions can make asthma worse. Ozone in the upper atmosphere protects us against the harmful rays of the sun. CFC *propellants* are contained in some asthma inhalers and contribute to the destruction of our protective ozone level; eventually these will all be replaced by a propellant that is safer for our environment.

Indoor pollution is as important a problem as that outdoors, and is mainly due to tobacco smoke, perfumes, aerosol sprays and, occasionally, inefficient gas fires. There is no doubt that all these substances can make asthma worse, and it is worth avoiding contact with them if at all possible. The problem, of course, is that we can have little control over the air that we breathe, except for tobacco smoke in the home.

> *TV weather forecasters talk about poor-quality air. Should I stay indoors or increase my treatment?*

It may be sensible to stay indoors when there is very poor air quality, but in some urban areas this might effectively put you under house arrest for long stretches of the year! Probably the most practical action you can take is to increase your *preventer* (inhaled steroids) treatment during these periods. If your symptoms are still uncontrolled, you might also need to start a short course of steroid tablets – all depending on your asthma action plan agreed with your doctor or asthma nurse. Poor air quality has been highlighted as a cause of worsening asthma control in certain individuals. As with people whose asthma is made worse by pollen, it can be very difficult to avoid the trigger of poor air quality.

The amount and quality of information gathered about air pollution will improve greatly in the coming years, and we will all become much more aware of the day-to-day changes in our atmosphere. Information about air quality and pollen are published in the newspapers and broadcast on the radio.

FOOD AND DRINK

Are certain foods unsuitable for people with asthma?

S omeone who has definite proven food allergy and also has asthma is at risk of having a life-threatening attack. However, true food allergy is not very common. Food allergy certainly exists and, when it is confirmed, may lead to severe asthma attacks and *anaphylaxis*.

Food allergy is more likely to occur in people who have other allergic conditions, such as a skin allergy called *urticaria*, and those whose asthma is triggered by, for example, dust, pollens and animals. Therefore someone who has both food allergy (confirmed) and asthma should ideally be under the care of an asthma specialist.

Sometimes, asthma triggered by food allergy may take several hours to develop, and so food might not be identified as the cause.

The most common food substances to cause asthma symptoms are cow's milk, nuts, peanuts, soft fruit (kiwi fruit, for example), shellfish, fish and yeast products. Food and drink additives can also cause asthma – see the answer to the next question for more details.

If you identify a food or drink that definitely makes you wheezy, it is sensible to avoid it wherever possible. If you suffer severely, and have had anaphylactic attacks from certain foods, you should be extremely careful to check ingredients in food you buy and eat. It is also important to understand that it is unlikely that food will be the only trigger. Sometimes, virus infections plus exposure to foods (or other allergens) may work in combination to cause an asthma attack. So it may be difficult to pinpoint the exact cause; if you think you have a food allergy, discuss this with your doctor. The condition should be confirmed by a specialist and, if necessary, you would be prescribed a self-injector adrenaline (epinephrine) syringe to use in an emergency.

Are food additives bad for people with asthma?

Some of them can be. Tartrazine (E numbers 102–110 and 210–219) is the most common additive causing problems for people with asthma. This is a yellow colouring that used to be found in many sweets and soft drinks, although more and more often now it is being omitted.

Food additives are marked on the labels of food containers in many countries. We advise that people with asthma should avoid tartrazine in particular. Other additives may also trigger asthma, but they may be very difficult to identify. Sodium metabisulphate and sulphur dioxide (SO_2), which are often contained in fizzy drinks, are other examples.

THE LONG-TERM OUTLOOK

Does good control of symptoms make the long-term outlook better for me?

Good control of asthma reduces symptoms, making a person feel better. Very often, people are unaware of how much they are tolerating asthma symptoms; when effective treatment removes these, they suddenly feel dramatically better. Thus there is no doubt that 'quality of life' is improved by good control of symptoms. There is also good evidence that effective control of asthma symptoms reduces the number of acute attacks.

These benefits are to do with the short-term outlook – in the next few years – for someone with asthma. We cannot say for sure yet that the outcome in 15, 20 or 30 years will be improved by good asthma control. We believe that it will be, but the research studies to prove or disprove it will take many years to complete.

In the meantime, we feel sure that the short- and medium-term benefits of good asthma control are sufficient to justify regular treatment as long as it is effective.

As I get older, will my asthma get worse?

This depends on how old you are when you ask this question! It used to be thought that nearly all children 'grew out of' their asthma by the end of their teens. Research has now found that this is not necessarily the case and only about one in three people lose their asthma completely. A further third either have a great reduction in symptoms or their asthma stops only temporarily. The other third continue to suffer from asthma, although often in a milder form.

In adults, the longer the asthma has been present, the more likely it is to have caused some permanent damage to the airways. In general, asthma can get worse as a person gets older, although even in adults asthma can improve or even disappear for many years.

There are other factors involved in getting older that may make asthma seem worse. Lung function decreases with age in everybody, so we have less in reserve when we require extra air. Other conditions such as chronic *bronchitis* and *emphysema* also become more common with increasing age, increasing the problems posed by asthma.

The best way to prevent asthma from becoming worse with age is to:

- avoid (or stop) smoking
- take preventer treatment regularly
- treat acute episodes early
- follow your agreed personal asthma action plan
- maintain general health and fitness as much as possible.

Will I need to be on oxygen when I get older?

This is very unlikely unless you have very severe, long-standing asthma. Lung function in people with severe chronic asthma tends to become worse and worse as the years go by. In such circumstances, oxygen in the home ('domiciliary oxygen') may be needed. This is provided under the direction of a hospital specialist or a specialist respiratory nurse.

If you do need oxygen at home a piece of equipment, called an oxygen concentrator, can extract oxygen from the air. The equipment is used with a facemask or nose tubing.

Sometimes, during severe asthma attacks, high doses of oxygen will be needed for a short time, but only to relieve the symptoms of the attack more rapidly. This will usually be part of the treatment provided by your doctor or hospital emergency department.

Personal action plan – things you might wish to discuss with your doctor or nurse

If, from time to time, you want to adjust your asthma medicines yourself, you will need a personal asthma action plan (self-management plan) from your doctor or nurse.

- A peak flow chart may help you to check your asthma.

- If you might have asthma that is aggravated or caused by exposure at work, you may need referral to a specialist in occupational medicine.

- If you are due to travel, make sure you that have an action plan, spare asthma medicines and information on the health services at your destination in case your asthma is troublesome.

- If you think food may be triggering your asthma, discuss this with your doctor. You might need food allergy tests, and you might need an adrenaline (epinephrine) injection to carry round with you.

- If you are allergic to a particular drug or substance, it would be worth considering registering for an 'alert' bracelet, necklace or wristband, so that emergency services can quickly identify possible problems if you suddenly become unwell. This allergy information can be very useful and, in some situations, life-saving.

7 | Children and asthma

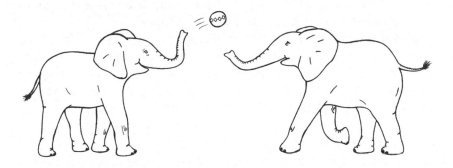

In this chapter you will learn about:

- asthma in infants and children

- useful tips to help you give asthma inhalers to infants and toddlers

- asthma at school, and the use of inhalers to promote independence

- potential side-effects of asthma medicines, and their safety

- asthma triggers

- the benefits of exercise

- asthma in adolescents.

Asthma is the most common *chronic* medical condition affecting children. We know that the number of children in the population who suffer from asthma has been increasing over the last 10 years, throughout the world. In an average primary school class there will be at least one child who has asthma and is receiving treatment for the condition.

Many children with asthma are still not always diagnosed with the condition, and therefore are not treated. They are just thought to be 'chesty' or to have repeated episodes of bronchitis. However, with increasing knowledge about asthma in childhood, more and more children are now correctly labelled as 'asthmatic'.

If a child's asthma is not correctly diagnosed and treated, he or she will suffer unnecessarily from respiratory symptoms and restraints in lifestyle such as loss of days at school and missing out on many social activities, both at home and at school. If asthma is not treated appropriately, the child will be at greater risk of becoming obese and less fit. The days when children with asthma were regarded as 'delicate' and 'highly strung' should be long gone. Many of the answers we give provide reassurance that it is possible for children to have a normal lifestyle.

In this chapter we discuss asthma across the spectrum of childhood, from infancy to adolescence. Asthma in infancy is often difficult to diagnose and treat, and presents a number of issues for children, parents and health professionals alike.

Asthma in early childhood varies widely, from occasional symptoms that occur only with coughs and colds (viral infections) to more persistent and troublesome symptoms, often related to allergic triggers or exercise. Some children seem to 'grow out' of their asthma as they get older, whereas in others the asthma persists into adulthood.

HOW AND WHEN DOES ASTHMA START?

Is asthma seen even in children less than a year old?

Yes, asthma can be seen in children under 1 year old but, at that age, there are other, more serious, diseases that can present with symptoms that mimic those of asthma. Also it is very difficult to diagnose asthma in very young children. It is important that these are considered and not missed. Any child who has frequent respiratory symptoms in the first year of life, such as wheezing or coughing that persists for weeks, should be referred to a specialist in childhood chest problems to find the cause of the problems.

Of great importance is the *family history*. If it includes asthma or other allergic diseases such as *eczema* or *hay fever*, the diagnosis of asthma is more likely in a child who gets lots of chest symptoms. In addition, children living in a house with a smoker are also more likely to develop asthma.

A detailed medical history is also of great help in confirming the diagnosis of asthma. The medical history includes information about:

- when the chest problems first appeared
- what sets off (triggers) the symptoms
- how frequently the symptoms appear
- whether they get better after a particular treatment.

However, in very young children the diagnosis is difficult to confirm because the required special tests can be done only in specialist children's facilities.

In very young children there are some clues to the diagnosis of asthma. These are children who:

- cough a lot, especially at night
- wheeze from time to time, especially with colds
- get colds that go to the chest and take several weeks to get better
- have persistent symptoms of cough and wheeze even when they do not have colds
- cough, wheeze or get chest tightness when they get excited or run around
- get better after anti-asthma treatment.

The doctor thinks my baby son has asthma. Why can't they do any tests so they can tell me definitely what the problem is?

As we say in the previous answer, there are no tests to confirm the diagnosis of asthma in babies and very young children, except in specialist children's hospitals. These tests may be used only in research projects.

Peak flow tests (see the sections on *peak expiratory flow* in Chapters 3 and 5) can be used at a later stage to confirm the diagnosis of asthma but this may not be feasible until your child is older than 5 years. The tests involve taking some readings using a peak flow meter or by more specialised blowing tests using equipment called a spirometer, but it can be difficult to obtain good test results in younger children unless the doctors or nurses are expert in carrying them out in children. In your baby's situation these tests are not feasible.

For your baby son, the diagnosis of asthma will be made after the doctor has examined him and asked you lots of questions. You will also be asked about your own health and that of other members of the family, because a *family history* of asthma makes the diagnosis of asthma more likely for your son. Putting all this information together will help the doctor come to a decision as to the likelihood of an asthma diagnosis.

It is frustrating for you if the doctor says he thinks your baby son has asthma because you want to know definitely, but this is not always possible. If the doctor thinks that your son has asthma, your son is likely to be prescribed anti-asthma medicines to see if they help. If they do help, it is very likely that your son does indeed have asthma.

Our child has asthma – whose fault is it? There is no history of it in our family.

Without knowing the precise circumstances we cannot be sure, but it would be wrong to 'blame' somebody for the development of asthma in your child.

Many children with asthma have a *family history* of asthma, *eczema* or *allergy* (e.g. house dust mite allergy or *hay fever*). These children inherit the asthma tendency in their genes. The asthma may show itself only when the child comes into contact with the relevant trigger factor such as dust or cats, or with exercise or a cold. Some children develop asthma even though no one else in the immediate family has it, but there is usually some asthma, hay fever or eczema on one or other side of the family.

My dad lives with us and smokes. I'm worried about my daughter because she is always coughing. I'm sure the smoke is making her worse. How can I get him to stop smoking?

There is a connection between smoking and respiratory symptoms in children. A child who is exposed to cigarette smoke in early life (while in the womb and during the first few years after birth) is at greater risk of developing asthma. Reducing exposure to tobacco smoke is sensible, and adopting a non smoking policy in the home is ideal but not always possible.

Passive smoking is a known trigger of asthma symptoms in people with the condition. The issue of smoking is a sensitive one, but do talk to your dad about your concerns. We are sure he doesn't want his grandchild to be troubled by his smoking, but it is a very addictive habit and is very difficult to stop. He may want to stop smoking but not know how or what help is available. Wanting to stop is the first stage of quitting smoking. Why don't you suggest that he talk to his doctor, practice nurse or local pharmacist about what help is available? There are many very effective smoking-cessation support programmes in place, which may help your dad.

If he does not want to stop smoking, ask him either to smoke outside or at least not in the same room as your daughter and the rest of the family. The problem is that the smoke clings to clothing and your child will still be affected by the smell of the smoke particles when he comes into the house. There are, of course, health and financial benefits to stopping smoking for your father, but he probably knows that. Try to be supportive and encouraging if he attempts to stop smoking and is unsuccessful. Many people do not succeed at their first attempt. It's always worth trying again!

My child wants a cat – do I go ahead and get him one, even though he has asthma?

Unfortunately, we cannot give a definitive answer and cannot tell you for sure if your child's asthma may be made worse. If you know that he is sensitive to certain animals, his asthma is likely to be worse if they live in your home. Having pets to which your child is allergic is not a good idea.

Children who live with a lot of animals such as those living on farms seem less likely to develop allergies but research has not proved this beyond doubt. The thinking behind this theory is that, when people are in contact with allergens (substances that cause allergy, such as cats, dogs, pollen, dust mites or certain infections), they develop *antibodies* to them. The antibodies can then work either to protect against disease or to actually cause disease if the person is exposed to larger quantities of those allergens. Whether a child develops asthma depends on two things: whether the child is allergic, and how much allergen they come in contact with.

This whole situation regarding pet ownership and asthma is very unclear. At the time of writing this book, it is not clear whether pet ownership definitely protects children against developing asthma or if pets are a cause of asthma. From the current research information we would not advise getting rid of animals if children are born into pet-owning homes. If the child (or someone else in the family) develops an allergy, you will need to decide whether to find a new home for the family pet. It would be worth discussing this with a health professional.

It might be sensible to get your child to stay with friends or relatives who have a cat and see if he reacts at all; it would be highly stressful for you, your child and the cat if you had to have it removed once it had become part of your family. However, be warned that people can be allergic to an individual animal and we would certainly advise you not to get a long haired type!

Is asthma more common in boys or in girls?

Childhood asthma is undoubtedly more common in boys. The reasons for the difference are not clear, and there does not seem to be any difference in the nature or severity of asthma.

The difference between boys and girls does not seem to be because of their different genetic makeup. There may be other factors earlier in childhood. For example, we know that boys have smaller airways as babies, and are more prone to respiratory infections than are girls. Boys are more likely than girls to 'lose' their asthma in adolescence. This also helps to explain how the ratios between boys and girls become more equal in adults.

My son is 7 years old. How can I find out how severe his asthma is?

The amount of treatment your son needs to control his asthma will give an indication as to how severe it is. It isn't always easy to judge the severity of your son's asthma because it may vary over time. Some children require more medication to control their asthma during the winter (more severe) than during the summer (mild asthma). Therefore, it is more relevant for you to assess whether your son's asthma is well controlled all the time (see Chapter 5 about asthma control and ways of assessing it). Regular assessment of your son's asthma control may also help you to adjust his controller (*preventer*) medication when the severity changes. That will reduce the risks associated with uncontrolled asthma (see 'Poor daily asthma control' in Chapter 2)

My son is 5 years old and has asthma. Is there any connection with the immunisations he has had?

No! There is no connection between routine childhood immunisations and asthma. These immunisations protect against potentially life-threatening disease and they do not cause or trigger asthma. Any chesty episode that occurs around the time of immunisation is purely coincidental.

Should I stop my child playing sport?

N o, not unless your child has been recently acutely unwell. It may be tempting for parents to stop their children from playing sport if this seems to bring on symptoms. Of course, if the asthma is in a bad phase and is out of control, it is sensible to do so, because exercise may make things get worse. However, the longer-term aim should be for good asthma control with *no limitations* on activities. Some of the best-known athletes and sports stars have asthma, and you may be hiding a potential Olympic champion!

Unfortunately, there are many children who have undiagnosed or uncontrolled asthma who give the appearance of disliking sporting activities. They may feel inadequate because their sporting performance is often poor when compared with that of their school friends. We often ask children with asthma what position they play on the soccer pitch, and 'goalkeeper' is a frequent answer. On closer questioning, we find that they may have chosen to play in goal because the position does not require too much exertion, and it therefore prevents any ridicule from their team-mates. A good test of asthma control is to ask the question again after they have received good asthma care. We have heard many times that, after effective treatment, they are able to play 'out' as well.

Remember that some children with asthma, on their own admission, use their asthma to get out of having to do sporting activities, even if it is not causing any problems at the time. Not all children enjoy playing sport, and in this respect children with asthma are no different from their peers.

INFANTS

When my 6-month-old daughter coughs a lot, should I give her cough mixture as well as her inhalers?

C oughing is a common symptom of asthma and, although it is tempting to use cough medicines, there is no evidence that they help. Many health professionals believe that cough mixtures are a waste of money! Using cough mixtures can create a false sense of security because you may think that no other treatment is needed. There are also possible dangerous side-effects from taking cough medicines, particularly if they contain codeine, which can have a harmful effect on breathing. Cough mixtures containing codeine or similar compounds should be avoided in children and should *not* be given to children under 1 year of age. It is best to use the asthma medicines as advised by the doctor or asthma nurse, and to seek help if they don't work.

One of the main problems in an infant of this age is actually getting the asthma medicines into the lungs. Young children often do not like inhalations through a facemask and inhalers, and it requires a lot of patience to get them to accept these devices. Once the device is tolerated, the medicines have a better chance of working and the symptoms will often disappear.

Are children who suffer from croup in infancy more at risk of developing asthma?

No. Croup causes narrowing of the larynx (voice box) and upper part of the trachea (windpipe) and, in this age group, is caused by respiratory virus infections (e.g. the common cold). Croup in infants and younger children results in a painful, barking cough and difficulty in breathing. It often affects the same child on a number of occasions, but it is a separate condition from asthma, and does not put the child at any increased risk of developing asthma.

Do I hold my baby down if she is fighting the facemask of her spacer device?

We believe you should never hold your child down to give her the asthma medicines. It can be really difficult to get young children to accept a facemask and spacer, and it requires a lot of patience on your part, especially if she is chesty and you are worried.

Although we normally say there must be a good seal between the mask and around the nose and mouth, if your daughter is very wheezy or breathless and is fighting the facemask, try holding the facemask a little distance away from her face. This is sometimes enough for a little of the medicine to be sucked in as she breathes, giving some relief. Once the airways start to open, babies often start to relax more, and will accept the mask more readily.

When your daughter is well, try to get her used to the spacer device and mask. Make it as much fun as you can, and very much a game. If she refuses the device or starts to get upset, put it away and try again later. Gradually your daughter will come to accept the device but it will take time and patience. If you get upset, so will she. Sometimes involving other people to give her the inhaler device, such as nursery staff, can be helpful. Giving her the asthma inhalers when she is not too tired and irritable may also be helpful. If your child has an older sibling, try letting the sibling inhale through the inhaler and face-mask (without releasing any medication). Younger children often want to copy the older children and therefore become much more interested in the inhaler. You can also give your daughter the inhaler and facemask to play with to familiarise her with the inhaler.

There are several different types of facemasks and spacer devices, and some may be accepted more readily than others. Sometimes a smaller device with a facemask or one that is brightly coloured is more acceptable than the larger spacers, but this is not always the case. Don't be tempted to give her the inhaler device when she is asleep. If she wakes up with a mask over her face, this may upset and frighten her.

Will giving inhalers to a baby prevent asthma from developing?

It is not possible to tell which babies will develop asthma in the future, and there is no justification for giving anti-asthma treatment before the condition has developed.

At present the main reason for prescribing inhaled asthma treatment is to control and reduce respiratory symptoms owing to asthma. Another reason is as a 'therapeutic test' – to see if the child gets better with asthma treatment; this frequently helps in making the diagnosis. Early treatment of asthma will shorten the duration of asthma symptoms, but the treatment cannot cure the asthma.

My 10-month-old baby recently saw a specialist because he gets very wheezy when he has a cold. The specialist mentioned viral wheezing one minute and then baby and infant asthma. I'm confused. What did he mean?

These terms are confusing, but they are all used to describe wheezing illnesses in young children. Virus infections are the most common trigger of asthma, and in young children they trigger wheezing and other respiratory symptoms such as coughing. At 10 months it is sometimes very difficult to say for sure whether your baby has asthma, because there are no easily applied tests to confirm the diagnosis, so these terms are used. Your specialist will have asked you lots of questions such as when the wheezing started, what sets it off, if there is a family history of asthma or hay fever, whether anyone smokes in the family and so on. The specialist will piece this information together to decide what the problem is most likely to be, because he will want to make sure that the wheezing is not a result of other conditions.

When the specialist has used the terms 'viral wheezing', 'baby asthma' and 'infant asthma' you can be happy that apparently there is nothing more serious going on. The specialist may recommend a trial of asthma inhaler treatments to see if they help relieve the wheezing symptoms. At your baby's age they are not always effective, because getting the asthma medicines into him can be quite difficult, even if a spacer device and facemask are used.

Inhalers are preferred to asthma syrup medicines because smaller doses of medicine can be given, but asthma syrup is still prescribed sometimes.

The other good news is that children who get wheezy in early childhood as a result of viral infections, but who have no family history of asthma (or other associated conditions), do seem to grow out of their symptoms as they get older.

CHILDHOOD

Does vomiting set off attacks of asthma in children?

No, vomiting doesn't set off an asthma attack in children; it is more likely to be the result of the asthma. Vomiting is quite common in young children with asthma who are troubled by frequent coughing.

Frequent coughing, especially at night, is a sign that the asthma is not under control. In young children, mucus from sore (inflamed) airways is usually swallowed because they do not spit it out. Pressure from distended lungs and coughing may squeeze the stomach, leading to vomiting.

The vomit contains lots of mucus (slimy phlegm). Children usually feel much better after they have vomited. If a child's asthma is not under control and they are coughing and vomiting, additional asthma treatment is usually needed.

Is it safe to let my 8-year-old decide how much Ventolin to take when she is away from me?

Yes it is, but it will depend on your child, her understanding and her physical capabilities: 8-year-old children can be very good at managing their own asthma, and can often stick to simple instructions. Most will be able to understand that they should take their reliever medication (Ventolin; salbutamol or albuterol) when they get asthma symptoms, as well as taking it before exercise in order to prevent getting exercise-induced symptoms. For these children it seems perfectly reasonable that they be allowed to decide when to take the Ventolin.

It is important to remember that, even if a child takes more than their usual dose of Ventolin inhaler, it will not do them any harm apart from increasing their pulse rate for a short time, and making them feel rather trembly. Children do not like these side-effects and therefore normally do not overdose with Ventolin.

If your daughter is using more and more Ventolin than usual and it doesn't seem to make any difference to her asthma symptoms, this is a sign that her asthma is getting worse. Your daughter needs to know that, if there are problems, she must get help from a grown-up or ask one of her friends to fetch help. You will need to make sure your daughter knows:

- what her reliever inhaler does
- when she should take it
- how much reliever to take each time
- what to do if it doesn't work
- when she can repeat the dose
- what to do if it still doesn't work, and how to get help.

Make sure your daughter's school has this information written down and also whom to contact if the Ventolin does not help her sufficiently.

One of the main problems for children occurs if they have an inhaler device that they cannot use very well on their own.

Metered-dose inhalers (spray inhalers) are difficult to use for people of all ages. Therefore, make sure that your daughter is capable of using her inhaler correctly every time she needs it. If you are not sure that she can, talk to your doctor about getting another inhaler or a spacer device for her spray inhaler (see Chapter 4 for more information about inhalers).

A dry-powder or a breath-activated inhaler is easier for your daughter to use when she is away from home, but these too may be difficult to use if asthma symptoms are very severe.

An inhaler that makes it easy to check how much Ventolin (salbutamol) your daughter uses is best, because then you can monitor how much medicine she has taken and how much is left in the device.

Alternatively, there are other dry-powder devices containing salbutamol (which is the same active ingredient as Ventolin). See Chapter 4 for details of other devices.

My child's asthma is always troublesome. Could this cause him not to grow properly?

Uncontrolled asthma can certainly be responsible for poor growth in children. Children with bad asthma often have delayed puberty. This means that they are often shorter than their friends in their early teens, but they do then 'catch up' in their late teens.

Growth hormone, which stimulates growth in the young body, is normally released in bursts during sleep and also during vigorous exercise. If your child does not sleep well or is unable to play sports because of poor asthma control, less of his growth hormone will be released. Children with severe asthma also tend be underweight because they have much higher energy requirements than normal.

Your child may need reassurance that he will grow taller. He may be quite sensitive about his lack of height in comparison with some of his friends. There is a wide variety in what is 'normal', and reassurance may be all that is required. Make sure that you talk to him about any concerns he may have, and ask that his height is checked at least 6-monthly or whenever you attend for an asthma review. If his height is plotted on a special growth chart, you and your son can check what progress there is. If you still have concerns about his lack of height, do talk to his doctor or asthma nurse, and they may refer you to a growth specialist for advice.

Is there any chance that I might give my child an overdose of her asthma treatment?

Asthma medicines are safe if they are given at the recommended doses, and overdoses are unlikely. The risks from asthma that is not sufficiently controlled are normally greater than the risks of the medications used for treating asthma. High doses of the *reliever* medicines (such as salbutamol (Ventolin) or terbutaline (Bricanyl)) may be life-saving in acute asthma situations. Giving 10–20 puffs or doses from a salbutamol inhaler may result in unpleasant side-effects such as a fast heart rate and trembling but these effects are not dangerous or long lasting. It is always important to seek urgent medical help if high doses of reliever medicines are needed. Additional medicines, such as a short course of prednisolone tablets or inhaled steroids, will be needed to gain control of asthma symptoms. Always seek help if your child's asthma fails to get better after the usual treatment.

Inhaled steroids (*preventers*) have a recommended upper dose limit. Your doctor or asthma nurse will plan with you the dose that your child should take. That will ensure that your child will only be prescribed a dose that will have fewer adverse effects on your child than the asthma itself will.

Leukotriene receptor antagonists (LTRAs; e.g. Singulair or montelukast) are chewable tablets. Side-effects are usually minimal but they may occasionally cause tummy aches or headaches.

There are no known risks of overdose with sodium cromoglicate (Intal) or nedocromil (Tilade). However, these drugs are not as effective as inhaled steroids and do not protect so well against asthma attacks.

It is possible to overdose people with the *theophylline* group of medicines such as aminophylline, theophylline (Nuelin) or theophylline (Slo-Phyllin). However, these are not used so often now because other asthma medicines are available that are usually more effective. If theophylline medicines are taken, they should always be used with caution and it may be necessary to have occasional blood tests to make sure that the blood levels are not too high.

In summary, asthma treatments are safe and effective when used at the correct dose to control symptoms. Asthma medicines should be reviewed at each asthma review with your child's doctor or asthma nurse.

How old does a child have to be before he can be skin-prick tested for allergies?

Skin-prick tests can be carried out at any age, even on a newborn baby. They are painless when carried out by an experienced person. A negative test on the skin does not prove that a child does not react internally to an allergen. A positive test is a bit more helpful, in that it does confirm the presence of the some allergy or allergic tendency (*atopy*) but it does not confirm the diagnosis of asthma.

Skin tests may be helpful if you want to check whether your child is allergic to, for example, cats. A positive cat-allergy skin test may help you make the decision against having a cat.

My child has asthma – how can I help make her lungs stronger?

Although it may seem surprising, your daughter's lungs are not necessarily any weaker than those of a child who does not have asthma. If asthma is controlled by giving the correct asthma medicines, which reduce the inflammation in the airways, the lungs will function absolutely normally. The best way for you to help your daughter is for you to encourage her to lead a full and active life with as few restrictions as possible. In this respect, physical exercise is very important.

In the few children with very severe asthma, special breathing exercises, taught by physiotherapists, may be necessary to improve the function of the lungs. However, these exercises are no more effective than regular physical exercise, so the latter is preferable if your child can do it. Talk to your doctor or asthma nurse if your daughter is in this group of children with very severe asthma.

Can a child with asthma be underweight?

Children with severe or poorly controlled asthma are quite often underweight. If there is a long delay in diagnosing their asthma, children may be underweight but then improve considerably once treatment is started.

Research has been carried out into the calorie intake needed for growth in children with poorly controlled asthma. Failure to thrive in childhood may have something to do with the extra effort required for day-to-day living with uncontrolled asthma. During acute asthma attacks, children may also use large amounts of energy.

Once the asthma is well controlled with the right treatment, children can catch up rapidly in terms of weight and growth. We have seen children who were underweight with poorly controlled asthma but who have improved dramatically once their asthma comes under control.

In a similar way, poorly controlled asthma may result in a child failing to gain height, as well as weight. Although there are concerns that high doses of steroid treatment may affect growth, it is more often the asthma that affects growth rather than the treatment. Make sure that your doctor or asthma nurse checks your child's height and weight at the asthma review. This can be recorded and any changes followed closely.

AT SCHOOL

In the United Kingdom, there is a statutory duty for governing bodies of maintained schools, proprietors of academies and management committees of pupil referral units (PRUs) to ensure their schools develop a policy for supporting pupils with medical conditions, such as asthma. This includes maintaining an individual health care plan for each of these children. In children with asthma, the plan must contain information on the child's triggers, as well as danger signs, symptoms and treatment. Details of what should be included in these plans is detailed on pages 77 to 100 and 156 of this book and in the national asthma guideline.

Should I tell a teacher that I have asthma?

Yes. It is important for your teachers to know about any health issues that may interfere with your schooling. If your teachers know about your asthma, they may be able to modify, for example, the science experiments or sporting activities so that you will not be affected by possible ill-effects – which can be quite common. Unfortunately, our experience is that teachers are often unaware that a pupil has asthma and so aren't sensitive to her or his needs.

Various school packs and school asthma cards have been developed to inform teachers about asthma and its treatment. Ask your doctor or asthma nurse about what is available in your area or if they know any good internet sites where this information is available. You may also find that your school has developed guidance for teachers about helping pupils cope with their needs, so it is important for your teacher to know about your asthma.

My teachers don't like me to use my inhalers at school. Is it all right to miss my lunchtime dose?

It is always best to take your asthma treatment as prescribed by your doctor or asthma nurse, but we are not sure what you mean by your lunchtime dose! Nowadays, *preventer* asthma medicines are taken twice or even once a day. If you are taking your preventer asthma inhalers more often, you should ask your doctor or hospital clinic about your treatment.

The usual asthma inhaler that you need to carry around with you is your blue *reliever* inhaler. Generally this is used 'as needed' but, if your asthma has been troublesome or you have a cold, you may need to use it more often. This can happen at school and it is important that you are allowed to use your inhaler if this occurs. If you are breathless, wheezy, coughing a lot or have chest tightness, you must use your blue reliever inhaler. You may also need to use your reliever inhaler before any sporting activities, to prevent exercise symptoms.

Unfortunately, some teachers do not realise the importance of taking reliever asthma treatment when it is needed. They may say that they find it disruptive to school routine if a child needs to use it. This may be because their school has a policy that requires all medicines, including asthma inhalers, to be locked away for safety purposes. For asthma, it would be far less disruptive if pupils with asthma had access to their inhalers at all times or were allowed to keep the inhaler with them. An inhaler is of no benefit if it is locked away and you are on a sports field or playground!

Perhaps you and your parents could speak to the school about the problems you are having. Alternatively, your doctor could ask the school nurse to discuss the issue of access to inhalers with the teachers at your school. Other possibilities are for your doctor to write to the school about the problem, or make contact with the school's parent governors or parent–teacher association. Sometimes the main problem is that people just don't know about asthma.

Can my son keep his inhaler with him in school?

As we have said in the previous answer, some schools have policies on whether or not children may keep their inhalers on them during school time. Unfortunately, some insist that all medicines be locked away, so that asthma treatments are inaccessible. Even if your son is not allowed to keep his inhaler in his pocket, he should have free access to it at all times. Delay in taking reliever treatment can lead to a severe attack.

Where possible, schools should discuss with the parents whether the inhalers are held by the pupil or by the school. For younger children, it seems sensible that the inhalers should be kept by the teacher in the classroom. For some older children at primary school, and for all those at secondary schools, the inhalers should be kept by the children themselves.

Why won't teachers give my daughter her inhaler?

This is quite a common problem. One of the difficulties for teachers is that the conditions of their employment do not include giving medicines or supervising a pupil to take them. However, our experience is that many are happy to supervise inhaler use but not make the decision to give it. Anyone taking on the responsibility of administering medicines should always have appropriate training and guidance.

In an emergency (e.g. an unexpected acute asthma attack – see Chapter 8), school staff are required to act as any reasonable or prudent parent would. This may include administering medication.

How can I convince other people (e.g. teachers) of the
seriousness of my child's condition?

If possible, try to arrange a time when you can talk with your
child's teacher. Unless you are absolutely sure of your facts, we
suggest that you take with you some reading material on the subject
of asthma and leave it behind for the teacher to read. You could also
take this opportunity to explain about the asthma medicines that
your child is taking, and the importance of making sure that they
are readily available when your child is at school. It may be worth
talking to the school nurse about any problems your child is having
at school.

Will teachers understand my son's asthma?

All surveys carried out to date show that school teachers have
only a limited understanding of asthma and its management.
Few teachers have received any training about the condition, and
they know little about the various treatments and the importance of
allowing children with asthma to keep their inhalers with them or
of the benefits of taking asthma treatment before games to prevent
asthma attacks.

If staff are ill-equipped to cope with children who have asthma,
they are more likely to be insecure and perhaps afraid of doing something wrong or even harmful to the child. (This can be regarded
by parents as a lack of interest by the teacher.) We feel that, with
increasing knowledge, teachers are becoming more confident about
coping with asthma. However, it will not be until all teacher training
colleges include sessions on asthma and all teachers receive guidance on the subject that the situation will be satisfactory.

What if another child at school gets hold of my daughter's
inhaler and uses it?

This is a common worry for both parents and teachers because
they fear that these medicines may be dangerous if given to the

wrong person. We can assure you, however, that no harm will come to a child who uses your daughter's inhaler – whatever treatment she takes.

Unfortunately, some children do sometimes use or play with metered-dose inhalers that belong to a child with asthma by spraying them around. This wastes the medicine and the real worry is that there won't be enough asthma inhaler medicine when your daughter needs it. If she is old enough to use a dry-powder inhaler, it is less likely that other children will use this device because it cannot be sprayed around and has to be put in the mouth to be activated. In any case, do speak to your child's teacher about your concerns.

GROWING OUT OF IT?

My 6-year-old son has asthma. Will he grow out of it?

This must be the most-asked question about asthma! Of course, everyone wants the answer to be 'yes' and it is very tempting to say that all children will grow out of their asthma. Unfortunately, this is not so. Without knowing more about your son's *medical history*, we cannot say for sure what will happen to him as he grows up. However, we do know that the milder the asthma, the more likely it is that the symptoms will disappear before he reaches adulthood. Some children seem to have their asthma symptoms (cough, wheeze and breathlessness) only when they have an *upper respiratory tract infection* (URTI; a cold or sore throat). For them the long-term outlook is also good. Finally, more boys than girls will grow out of their asthma before adulthood.

On the other hand, if the asthma is in association with an allergy such as *hay fever* and/or *eczema*, it is more likely that the symptoms will continue into adulthood. Sometimes the symptoms may lessen or disappear at puberty even in these children, but they frequently come back later in adult life. The earlier a child develops asthma and the more frequent and severe the attacks, the less chance there is of the asthma disappearing in adolescence. Even if the asthma disappears before adulthood, it may return later in adult life after several years without any symptoms. Therefore, it is important to remember that, once you have had asthma, you may always have an 'asthma tendency', and that the asthma can recur at any time.

> *I had asthma as a child but then I was free of it for many years. Why did it return in adulthood?*

The simple answer is that we don't know. It is well recognised that asthma can return after years of not having any symptoms at all (see the previous answer). This is why we tend to talk about asthma going 'into *remission*' rather than disappearing.

ADOLESCENTS AND YOUNG ADULTS

> *I read somewhere that children who have asthma mature later than average. Is this true?*

Research has found that children with asthma tend to mature physically 1–2 years later than other children, and the delay may be more marked in children with difficult asthma. This has been known for many years – even before the modern treatments were available; so changes in treatment do not seem to be the cause. X-rays of bones in children give a good indication of maturity and, in children with asthma, *bone age* will often be 1–2 years behind their actual age

The practical effect of this is most important in adolescents, as they will have their growth spurt and their signs of puberty later than their friends who do not have asthma. Although we can reassure them that they will 'catch up' later, this may be of little comfort at a time when it is so important to them to be the same as everybody else.

So, in physical terms it is true that children mature later, but there is no evidence that young people with asthma mature emotionally later than their peers.

Height and weight should be measured and recorded at each asthma review. This will enable the doctor or asthma nurse to monitor growth and reassure both the child and the parents. The delayed-growth issues need to be handled very sensitively, and concerns listened to and acknowledged.

I'm in the middle of my examinations and my asthma has got much worse because of the pressure. I'm afraid that I might have an attack during one of my papers. How can I prevent this?

All examinations cause stress, and some students cope better than others. As important school exams are held in the summer months, this brings added problems because they coincide with the hay fever season and high pollen counts. Both of these factors make asthma worse in many young people. Prevention wherever possible is always better than cure, and there are a few things that may help.

- Spring time is a good time to visit your doctor or asthma nurse for extra advice about your asthma control. Regular assessment (see Chapter 5) will help you find out whether your asthma is well controlled or not. If your asthma is not under good control, your asthma medicines need to be reviewed by your doctor or asthma nurse. Hay fever medicines may also reduce the trigger effect of pollen on the asthma.

- Always make sure that you carry your *reliever* inhaler with you, and take your *preventer* treatment as discussed with your doctor or asthma nurse. If you are already in the middle of your exams, and your asthma is not well controlled, you may want to ask them about a possible short course of steroid tablets to tide you over the most important exam days. If you suffer badly from your asthma or hay fever during the exam time and you feel this has had an effect on your exam performance, a certificate or letter from your doctor or asthma nurse stating the problems you have had may help the examiners.

- Despite your exams, make sure you have some time to enjoy a social life and activities with friends. This helps to relieve some of the tensions that you are all under and provides a good network of support. Relaxation can help to reduce the chances of having an asthma attack owing to stress.

- Ask your doctor or asthma nurse for a personal asthma action plan to help you know what to do if symptoms are troublesome. They will work out a plan with you that is right for you. This plan can be based on either asthma symptoms or control assessment.

Personal action plan – things you might wish to discuss with your doctor or asthma nurse

- How can I help keep my child's asthma under control?

- What do I do if my child's usual reliever inhaler is no longer effective?

- Can you tell me what to look for, so I know if my child is having an asthma attack?

- Will a peak flow meter be useful to check if my child's asthma is getting worse?

- How can I help my child if the asthma gets worse?

- After a bad asthma attack, does my child need to see the doctor or asthma nurse?

- Does my child need to see the doctor or asthma nurse for a regular check-up?

---

8 | Emergencies

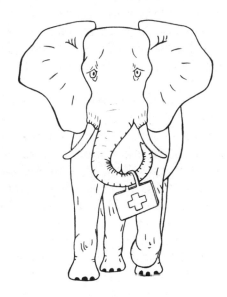

In this chapter you will learn:

- how to tell when your asthma is going out of control

- about the danger signs that may be present before an asthma attack

- when to worry and when to call for help

- what immediate action to take while waiting for help

- how to learn lessons from asthma attacks and how to prevent them in future.

Asthma can be well controlled in most people. However, it does go out of control at times and, if not dealt with rapidly, can lead to a medical emergency. This is important because uncontrolled asthma may lead to an asthma attack, which can be very serious. Sadly, asthma attacks can be fatal but many of these severe attacks can be prevented.

If health professionals as well as people with asthma (or their carers) can improve how they recognise the early warning signs, and if the right action is taken, many asthma attacks and hospital admissions can be prevented.

Throughout this book we stress the need to recognise uncontrolled asthma. Early action on your part to prevent the asthma episode from worsening is so important. The first section in this chapter deals with the early warning signs and symptoms of asthma attacks. The most important of these is the failure of symptoms to respond to your usual *reliever* treatment. If this happens to you, don't accept it as 'just one of those things'! It is a sign of potentially serious trouble and perhaps the beginning of an asthma attack.

The second section gives advice on what to do if you or someone you are with has an asthma attack. It can be important to get to hospital urgently. In this section you will learn when to call for an ambulance or make your way quickly to hospital, without first seeing your family doctor.

The decision to 'self-refer' to hospital rather than asking your doctor to refer you should be part of an agreed plan between you and the hospital specialist, doctor or nurse (see the section on 'Written personal action plans for asthma' in Chapter 5).

The final section of the chapter deals with recovery from asthma attacks. This is just as important as recognising the early stages. Everyone with asthma is more vulnerable and may suffer a repeat episode in the weeks or months following an attack. It is a time when you should take a very careful note of your symptoms and peak flow readings. Do go to your doctor or nurse for an asthma check as soon as possible after an acute attack. The main reason for this is to find out if the attack is over and if it could have been prevented. In particular, do you need more treatment for the attack; were you on the correct treatment for your asthma, and were you taking it in the right way?

If you are admitted to hospital, arrangements should be made for you to be seen again for a follow-up soon after you return home. This might mean that you will be seen for a check-up at the hospital or by your family doctor. In either event, you should ensure that you have a check-up within 2 days after the attack.

SYMPTOMS AND WARNINGS

What are the warning signs and symptoms of an asthma attack?

Most people have asthma symptoms, such as cough, wheeze or shortness of breath, for a number of days before they have an asthma attack. Sometimes these symptoms are present for a few weeks or even months without the person realising that they are due to the asthma being out of control.

Some people with asthma say that they do not feel they are listened to when they consult a doctor or nurse for their asthma. The reason for this may be that some health professionals are not sufficiently aware of the danger signs of asthma attacks. It may also be that the person with asthma does not explain clearly what they are worried about, or that they don't describe all their symptoms to the doctor or nurse.

It is therefore very important to explain that you think the symptoms may be due to uncontrolled asthma when you seek medical help in this situation. At the end of this chapter, we list some of the things you might want to discuss when you see your doctor or asthma nurse for check-ups.

Warning signs before an asthma attack vary from person to person. In one rare form of asthma, known as *brittle asthma*, people may go from no symptoms at all to severe, acute, life-threatening asthma within minutes. Sometimes this will happen due to an allergic reaction. For most people, however, there are clear warning signs. These include:

- your usual symptoms of asthma getting worse or going on for days

- you don't get your usual improvement from using your *reliever* inhaler

- changes in peak flow readings – if you monitor your own *peak expiratory flow*, changes in the readings are usually present before the symptoms start; these readings therefore give early warnings of an asthma attack. There are three patterns (also discussed in Chapter 3) to watch out for:
  - an increased difference between morning and evening readings
  - steadily falling readings
  - morning dips

- unusual symptoms, which often occur before an attack – examples of these are a tickly cough, a strange sensation in the skin (usually an itch – in children) or in your nose, light-headedness or sickness; there are other warning symptoms and it is important for everyone to recognise their own.

Asthma attacks vary from mild to very severe.

- Mild attacks may involve only slight coughing, wheezing or difficulty in breathing.

- In a severe attack, there will be extreme difficulty in speaking and breathing. A person may become blue (seen on the lips, in the lining of the mouth or fingernails) due to shortage of oxygen (*cyanosis*). They may have a very fast heart rate and complain of 'thumping' in the chest, and they may sit upright leaning on their outstretched arms (to support their chest). They may be very short of breath and gasping for air. The other thing that happens is the person's muscles in between the ribs pull inwards with breathing. If any of these things is happening, help the person by giving them their reliever inhaler (see Table 8.1) and calling for an ambulance urgently – say the person is having a severe asthma attack!

It is important to be aware that a mild attack can develop into a very severe one. This may occur suddenly or take a few days or weeks to happen. It is for this reason that *all asthma attacks should be taken seriously*, even if they seem to be mild. Furthermore, because attacks can occur in anyone with asthma, it is important to know how to deal with uncontrolled asthma. Relief from medication that doesn't last for 4 hours or doesn't have its usual effect is a very important sign, both for people with asthma and for health professionals. It is very important to tell your doctor or asthma nurse if your usual medication is not helping your asthma symptoms.

How do I tell if my asthma symptoms are serious?

The symptoms of an attack are the same as those of asthma itself – coughing, wheezing and difficulty in breathing.

All of these symptoms may occur together but, during an acute attack, shortness of breath is usually the most noticeable. If you suddenly get worse, your asthma symptoms should improve when extra relief (*reliever*) medication is taken. This improvement should last for at least 4 hours. Therefore, if your symptoms are getting worse and they do not improve with your usual asthma relief medication, or if they worsen again within 4 hours, you should seek urgent medical advice.

Someone whose asthma is well controlled should not be getting these symptoms. If you are, you probably need more or different asthma medicines. When you phone your doctor's practice, explain clearly to the receptionist what is happening. Say that your asthma is out of control and that you need to see the doctor or nurse urgently. When you reach the doctor's office, repeat all the information to the doctor or nurse, because the receptionist may not have done so.

'Everyone' seems to know how to treat an epileptic fit or diabetic emergency, but not how to treat someone having an asthma attack. Why? Is it the fault of first-aid courses which give it such a low priority? Should there be more public education?

Most courses on basic life support nowadays include the management of acute severe allergic reactions, called *anaphylaxis*. However, asthma has had a very low profile until recent years, and very little attention has been paid to teaching people how to cope with someone having an attack. As it is one of the most common medical conditions in the developed world, there definitely should be more public education about it. We certainly hope this will change as public recognition of the importance of asthma increases.

There are excellent sources of educational information from patient-orientated organisations dealing with asthma. For example: in the United Kingdom, Asthma UK; in Australia, the Asthma Foundation Australia; in Europe, EFA (European Federation of Allergy and Airways Diseases Patients Associations); in the United States, AAFA (Asthma and Allergy Foundation of America). The Global Initiative for Asthma (GINA) is a good resource if you want to read about the usual expected treatment of people with asthma. Contact details are given in the Useful Addresses appendix.

What is a 'silent chest'?

When someone has an attack, one or more of the common symptoms of asthma – coughing, wheezing and shortness of breath – increase. As long as air is passing in and out of the lungs, the wheezing will continue and can be heard, and the breathing will tend to be quite noisy. However, when the air passages are so tight that very little air can get into and out of the lungs, these symptoms are less obvious. In particular, there may be no wheezing, and in this case the breathing becomes very quiet. When the doctor or asthma nurse listens with a stethoscope, no sounds of breathing are heard.

This situation where someone is having difficulty getting air in and out of their lungs is described as a *silent chest*, and all doctors recognise it as a sign of a very severe attack. Emergency treatment is required.

FIRST AID FOR EMERGENCIES

If you are worried that your asthma attack is getting very bad or if you are worried about someone else who is having an attack, call for advice or help immediately. While waiting for help, it is important to ensure that the *reliever* medication is used – in high doses if necessary. Detailed information is given later in this chapter, but the essential points in dealing with asthma episodes follow.

If my chest feels very tight and my reliever – Ventolin (salbutamol) – is not working, what should I do?

F ailure to obtain relief from your usual reliever, whichever one you take (albuterol, salbutamol, terbutaline), is an important sign of uncontrolled asthma. An attack may be on the way, and quick action is needed. Seek medical advice urgently. In the meantime, self-treatment must be continued. Even though your reliever may not seem to be working, it is important to take it in high doses until you can get other treatment. Ideally, you will have discussed with your doctor or asthma nurse what to do if this situation arises, but the following will help as general guidance.

- Emergency use of reliever inhalers. Usually, 2–4 puffs, taken one puff at a time and inhaled separately, every 10–20 minutes is sufficient. However, if you are not getting relief, take extra puffs until the emergency services arrive. If you have a spacer device available (see Figure 4.15), use this to take the medication. If not, a simple paper coffee cup or paper rolled into a cone or a plastic bottle may be used (see Figure 8.1). This way of taking your reliever medicine works as well as a nebuliser (see Figure 4.17) and is perfectly safe when used in an emergency. Once you have taken your asthma reliever

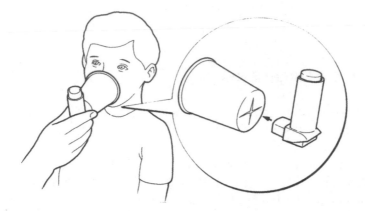

Figure 8.1
Makeshift spacer.
This is a paper cup
with a hole cut in
the bottom to fit
an inhaler device. A
rolled-up piece of
paper in the shape
of a funnel may
also be used in an
emergency.

EMERGENCY TREATMENT VIA THE SPACER DEVICE

1. Put 2 parts of the spacer device together.

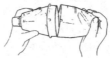

2. Remove the mouthpiece cap from the metered dose inhaler.

3. Shake inhaler and insert into flat end of spacer.

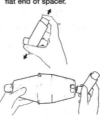

4. Place spacer mouthpiece in patient's mouth and press inhaler canister once to release a dose of the short acting bronchodilator medication. (If unable to use the mouthpiece, attach facemask to the mouthpiece end and place over nose and mouth ensuring a good seal.)

5. Only one dose of medication should be actuated at a time.
6. Ask the patient to breathe in and out through the spacer device for 4 or 5 breaths.
7. Remove mouthpiece from patient's mouth.
8. For effective relief of symptoms in acute asthma repeat steps 4–7. Up to 20 puffs (actuations) of a short acting bronchodilator may be required for adult patients (up to 10 puffs for children).
9. Shake the inhaler canister gently between actuations. This can be done with the canister still inserted in the spacer device.

If there is no immediate improvement or the patient's condition continues to deteriorate, seek urgent medical help. Whilst waiting for emergency assistance repeat above steps.

medicine, concentrate on breathing steadily and staying relaxed. It is still important to call for help or advice, even if you feel better.

- Steroid tablets. Most asthma guidelines also recommend that you start taking steroid tablets (prednisolone) straight away if you have them available. This should be part of your action or self-management plan; if not, we suggest that you discuss it with your doctor. A dose of 30–60 mg (6–12 tablets) for adults and 20–30 mg (4–6 tablets) for children is usually suitable. These tablets take up to 6 hours to start working and you will need to take them for several days until the attack is over.

What is the best way for me to treat a very bad attack?

During a very bad attack it becomes difficult for you to speak, because of breathlessness. This is an emergency, which needs treatment in hospital. On the way or while you are waiting for medical help, take a high dose of *reliever* medication: usually 6–10 puffs, taken one at a time, and inhaled separately preferably via a spacer, every 10–20 minutes. Sometimes higher doses are needed and it is important to take more reliever medicine if you do not improve at all. These doses are not dangerous; in fact the equivalent of 25–50 puffs of Ventolin (albuterol, salbutamol) is the dose that is given in a nebuliser. If you have a spacer device available, use it to take your reliever.

Table 8.1 lists some advice about recognising a severe asthma attack and some first-aid treatment while waiting for medical assistance to arrive.

Table 8.1 Emergency treatment for a severe attack

Use a spacer device if one is available.

Any of these signs means the attack is severe

1. The usual reliever medication does not help (it should work immediately and should last for 4 hours).

2. The symptoms (cough, breathlessness, wheeze or whistling sounds from the chest) get worse.

3. The person is too breathless to speak normally.

How to deal with the attack

1. Give the reliever drug (6–10 puffs, one at a time).

2. Call the doctor or ambulance if the condition is not relieved in 5 minutes. If the attack is very bad, call for medical help immediately.

3. If the person has an emergency supply of oral steroids (cortisone, prednisolone; soluble prednisolone), give the stated dose as soon as possible.

If you don't have a spacer device with you, you could use a make-shift spacer by adapting a paper coffee cup or a piece of paper rolled into a cone shape, as shown in Figure 8.1. Otherwise, use your reliever device as best you can, as often as you need until you feel better or until emergency help arrives.

Salbutamol or terbutaline should start to work within a few minutes and this is why it is *always* important to carry your reliever treatment with you. If your peak flow meter is available, take a peak expiratory flow reading before you start and make a note of the result. Check your peak flow again after about 15 minutes to see if it has improved. This way you can see if your reliever medicine is helping.

Try to remain calm, and arrange to get to hospital. If your own doctor is with you, he or she will arrange for an ambulance. If you are on your own, phone the emergency services and ask for an ambulance. Tell them your asthma is severe and that you need help urgently.

For an asthma attack, a course of steroid tablets is often necessary. If you have these available, the course should be started straight away as advised by your doctor. These tablets take approximately 6 hours to start to work, so it is important to start them as soon as possible, particularly if you are away from home and there may be some delay in getting medical attention. Steroid tablets save lives in severe asthma attacks, and they should be used early in the attack rather than as a last resort. It is important to discuss an action plan for your asthma with your own doctor or asthma nurse when you are well, so that you are confident about what to do if you have a bad attack.

Can I go straight to hospital if I have an attack?

Yes, you can – and it may be the best step for you to take if you suffer from sudden severe asthma attacks. If you are one of those few people whose asthma is bad enough to require several hospital admissions each year, you will probably be under specialist care – or should be. Usually you will have instructions as to when it is best to go direct to hospital.

For most people with asthma this is not the case, and most asthma attacks can be managed without the need for hospital admission. Your doctor and nurse are likely to be familiar with your asthma, and in a good position to help deal with acute attacks.

How do we know when to go to hospital?

In emergencies there are two options open to you for medical help.

- The first is to contact your general practice or family doctor, and this is what we would suggest in most situations.

- In certain circumstances it may be better to go straight to hospital. This applies to children as well as adults. If someone has had a number of admissions to hospital for acute asthma, it is best to agree with the specialist at the hospital what to do. This is called an 'open door policy', and it means that, if you or your child has a bad attack that is not responding to an agreed treatment plan, you can go direct to the hospital ward, without contacting your family doctor first.

Agreeing an 'open door policy' with the specialist is best for children who have repeated admissions for asthma, and for adults with *brittle asthma* whose attacks come on rapidly and can be very severe. For most other people with asthma, it is usually best to see a doctor or asthma nurse who knows you or your child's history.

Emergency care varies in different countries. So it's best for you to find out from your doctor what to do in emergencies. Family doctors in the UK's National Health Service provide emergency care during the working day; however, under fairly new arrangements, many do not do so after normal working hours. In most parts of the UK, emergency out-of-hours care is provided either by cooperatives run by local doctors or by primary care organisations. These 'Urgent Care Centres' are usually located in hospital grounds, but they don't often have equipment for treating severe asthma attacks. So if you or someone you are caring for is having a severe attack, go to the main hospital Accident and Emergency department!

During normal hours, your doctor will probably be able to manage most asthma attacks. However, if admission to hospital is needed, it is generally better for your doctor or nurse to arrange this and for you to go to the hospital with a referral letter from the practice – unless of course you are extremely unwell, when an ambulance is best. If your doctor cannot be contacted, it is safer to go straight to hospital.

Most asthma attacks may be prevented by taking regular asthma medicines as advised by the doctor or nurse, by having regular medical check-ups and by following an agreed personal asthma action plan.

When asthma is diagnosed, three important questions should be answered to your satisfaction by your doctor or asthma nurse:

- What should I do in an attack?

- How do I get medical help in an emergency?

- When should I go straight to the hospital?

If you haven't covered these questions with your doctor or nurse (or have forgotten the answers!), go over them when you next have the opportunity.

Most people's asthma is not so severe that immediate treatment at the hospital is required. It is much better for you to have guidance from your doctor before a problem arises, rather than afterwards.

Many people with uncontrolled asthma symptoms wait far too long before contacting their doctor. If your usual asthma medicine is not helping, or if you are getting increasing symptoms of cough, wheeze or shortness of breath, see or speak to your doctor or nurse as soon as you can.

In a severe attack, go to the hospital first.

Can a child die of asthma?

Sadly, yes, anyone can die from an asthma attack. In children, such tragedies are very rare but do occur. Accurate statistics are not readily available for all countries but here are a few. In 2012, in the UK, there were about 1200 deaths due to asthma, and 36 of these were in children. In Australia in 2011, there were 378 deaths due to asthma, and fewer than 20 of these were children.

Unfortunately, some asthma deaths cannot be prevented, but many have involved preventable or avoidable factors. These include both patient and doctor. In children, many asthma deaths result from sudden unexpected fatal attacks, nearly always against a background of very severe asthma or *allergy* (e.g. to peanut).

Anyone with a previously diagnosed severe food allergy *and* asthma should have an emergency kit available, in addition to the usual asthma medication. This kit includes a special adrenaline (epinephrine) injection for self-use (Epipen or Anapen), a course of steroid tablets and a course of antihistamine tablets.

A fatal asthma attack is exceptionally rare in a previously healthy child. We would like to be completely reassuring on this point, but tragedies do happen. People with asthma must always be cautious if an attack of asthma seems different in some way from previous episodes, or is unresponsive to reliever treatment.

What if I have an attack and I have no medication?

Ideally, this should not happen. Asthma attacks can occur without warning, so you should always have some *reliever* medication available, wherever you are. If, however, you have an attack and no medication is available, take steps to obtain treatment straight away, either from your doctor or pharmacist or from the nearest hospital if your symptoms are severe.

In the UK you are able to obtain an emergency supply of your asthma treatment from a local pharmacist. You will need to give some details about your asthma as well as pay for the medicines. You will pay the cost of the medicines and a dispensing fee, because the medicines are not being obtained on a prescription.

Obtaining your asthma medicines in this way is *only for exceptional situations*. You should take care not to run out of any regular medicines and should obtain a 'repeat' prescription before this happens. In many countries, including Scandinavia and the USA, these medications are available only with a doctor's prescription, even in an emergency.

If the attack occurs when you are away from home and in the UK, emergency treatment is available from any doctor working in the National Health Service. However, if you have a *severe attack*, we would always recommend hospital as the first choice. If you are in doubt about how severe your attack is (and it can be difficult to judge), always be on the safe side and seek advice about your asthma at the hospital.

Please take advice from your doctor if you are planning to travel abroad, and also ensure that you have enough medication, for emergencies as well as for regular use.

In an untreated attack, delay can be serious and on some occasions has been fatal. In some countries, it is possible to get a *reliever* inhaler (Ventolin, salbutamol or albuterol are well known) from a pharmacy, without a prescription. This will be helpful while finding local medical help.

My friend has asthma. What do I do if I am with her and she has an asthma attack?

I f your friend is distressed and having difficulty breathing, this is a potentially severe attack.

- Stay calm.

- First, as in the case of any medical emergency, call for someone to help. Call an ambulance immediately – or ask someone else to do so, if possible. Then you can start helping your friend.

- Ask her if she has her *reliever* inhaler (Ventolin, salbutamol or albuterol; or terbutaline) with her. If she has, help her to take large doses of the reliever inhaler as best she can – usually 2–6 puffs, taken one after the other. This can be repeated every 20–30 minutes (or more frequently if there is no effect). Tell her to take more if necessary while waiting for help to arrive.

- If she is struggling to use her inhaler, you can help her by making an emergency spacer device using a piece of paper rolled into a cone, or by making a hole in the bottom of a paper or polystyrene cup (see Figure 8.1). Hold the cone in front of her face, and fire the inhaler 2–6 times, one puff at a time, with about 10–15 seconds between each puff, so that she can breathe in the spray via the cone or cup. Use more if she is not improving, and repeat this every few minutes while waiting for help. It is safe to do this, and it will nearly always bring some temporary relief.

You won't be able to use a spacer or coffee cup for the dry powder devices, but you can give repeated doses without any risk of overdose.

Should I consult a doctor before administering Ventolin nebuliser to my son with asthma if he has an attack?

Because there are no dangers from using a single dose in this way, it is probably better that you start treatment immediately and then call the doctor or ambulance service, depending on the circumstances. This treatment may be life-saving in a severe attack.

The potential problem does not come from the nebuliser, or even from the medicine in the nebuliser. The danger comes from *not recognising* when asthma is getting worse, and from *not doing enough*. We would advise that a short course of steroid tablets is also needed whenever an attack is bad enough to need high doses of reliever treatment. So, even if your son is a lot better after the treatment, he should still see a doctor or asthma nurse urgently – within a few hours if possible.

If he needs a nebuliser for an attack, this is because his asthma is out of control. If the nebuliser relieves the symptoms for at least 4 hours, this indicates that his attack has responded to the treatment, and he should continue with his self-management (or action) plan.

However, if the attack does not respond, it is important that other treatment be obtained. We now know that a spacer device works as well as a nebuliser in most cases of acute asthma, so long as high doses of reliever medicine are used. Nevertheless, anyone having a severe attack is best treated in a hospital, so, after using the emergency treatment, it is advisable to get to a hospital.

My sister has asthma. How can I help her if she starts to hyperventilate?

You need to ensure that she really is hyperventilating. *Hyperventilation* (or over-breathing) means breathing more rapidly than is necessary or than is good for someone. It occurs commonly in people who are anxious or frightened (whatever the reason), and causes symptoms of light-headedness, feeling sick, and tingling in the hands and feet and around the lips. For someone with an asthma attack, who is trying desperately to breathe, it is an understandable reaction. Try to encourage her to slow down her breathing by taking 5–10 seconds to breathe in and 5–10 seconds to breathe out. Extra use of her *reliever* medication will help to improve the asthma attack and this, hopefully, should reduce her hyperventilation.

The well-known trick of breathing in and out of a paper bag is less helpful in asthma than in other circumstances. There is already a shortage of oxygen, and this may be made worse by breathing in used air from a bag. It will be more useful to talk slowly and reassuringly to your sister in order to slow down her rate of breathing.

For the future, relaxation exercises are good preparation for dealing with asthma attacks. Check the internet, your local library or with your family doctor for information on relaxation exercises.

How bad does an attack have to be before I seek medical advice?

Everyone's asthma is different, so the detailed answer to this question depends a lot on the features of your own asthma. Past experience is often helpful in deciding whether you need help. If you have ever been admitted to hospital with asthma, if you are obese, if your asthma is poorly controlled or if you are not good at remembering to take your inhalers, it would be best to see your doctor before a mild attack becomes a severe one.

Ideally, you and everyone else should have a personal action or self-management plan for treating asthma episodes (see the section 'Written action plans for asthma' in Chapter 5).

When your asthma goes out of control, you follow the plan. If your symptoms fail to improve, you need medical advice. Severe symptoms mean that you must call for medical help straight away. Below are some examples of severe symptoms:

- difficulty in speaking, or not being able to complete sentences in one breath

- severe difficulty in breathing

- blue discoloration of the lips or tongue

- a very fast pulse (more than 120 per minute in an adult or more than 140 per minute in a child)

- a very fast breathing rate (more than 25 per minute in an adult, more than 30 in children aged 5–15 years and more than 50 per minute in preschool children)

- becoming exhausted by the attack

- a peak flow reading less than half the usual level.

If you are unsure, it is always better and safer to seek advice early in an asthma attack, rather than later. The worse your asthma attack is when you ask for help, the more difficult it is to treat. (See also the information in the section 'Symptoms and warnings'.)

RECOVERY PERIOD

For how long do I need to continue a higher dose of my inhalers after I have had a cold?

This is another of those situations that are different for each person; there is no rule that will work for everyone. You are doing the right thing by increasing your medication when an important trigger factor, such as a cold, comes along. The trigger makes the airways hyperreactive (*bronchial hyperreactivity*), or 'twitchy', and this may lead to a bad attack of asthma. It is wise to try to prevent this by increasing the use of relief (*reliever*) medication as well as the *preventer* (if you usually take both of these).

A useful rule of thumb is to continue on the higher dose for 2 weeks after the episode has improved; then the dose of preventer can be reduced to your previous level. This method often works well but it is not always suitable for everyone.

There are three ways to tell if your asthma has settled down after an attack. The best way to tell if your asthma has improved after an attack is to keep a peak flow diary chart, which gives a more accurate picture of when the asthma episode is over. Figure 8.2 shows the chart of a boy whose asthma went out of control and then improved spontaneously. By using the chart it is possible to see when the peak flow readings have returned to the previous 'best' levels.

The action you take when your asthma goes out of control depends on the advice from your doctor, and agreed in your self-management plan. The idea of a personal asthma management plan is to help you recognise when to adjust your treatment, when it's safe to resume your normal treatment and when you should call for help. Having treated your attack and your symptoms and readings have settled at your normal level, and are not changing much from day to day, you can then reduce the dose and resume your normal treatment. If you continue to keep your diary, you will be able to tell when to increase your asthma medicines again if your condition deteriorates.

This approach ensures that you take sufficient medication when you need it and also that you do not take more than necessary. Figure 8.3 shows a peak flow chart where a boy has taken steroid

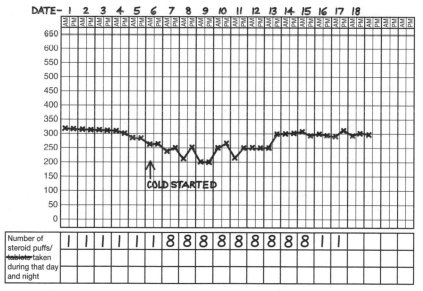

Figure 8.2 A peak flow chart of a boy whose asthma went out of control and then improved spontaneously.

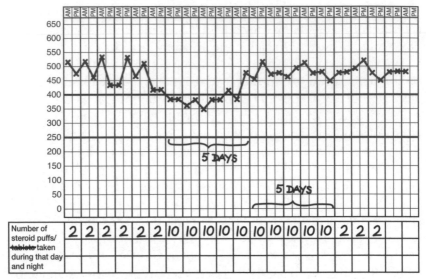

Figure 8.3 Peak flow chart of a boy with an asthma attack. He recognised that his peak flow readings were dropping, so he took steroid tablets (prednisolone) to prevent the attack from getting worse. He stopped the tablets when his readings were returning to normal

tablets (prednisolone) to treat an attack when his readings dropped and symptoms got worse.

We give more detail about using your chart to decide when it is safe to reduce your dose to its normal level in the section on 'Written action plans for asthma' in Chapter 5.

The other two ways to tell if your asthma has settled down are your ongoing need for reliever treatment, and your symptoms. If you still need to take more than four puffs of your reliever inhaler in a week, your asthma is poorly controlled. Similarly, if your symptoms of cough, wheeze or shortness of breath are continuing, your asthma is not yet controlled. If either of these is happening, it would be wise to see your doctor.

Personal action plan – things you might wish to discuss with your doctor or asthma nurse

In this chapter you learnt how to tell if you are going to have an asthma attack, what to do if your symptoms get worse or if you do have an attack, and what to do after an asthma attack or after an episode of uncontrolled asthma. The most important thing is that you should see your doctor or nurse for a check-up within 3 days of having an asthma attack.

When you go for this check-up, it will be helpful if you take your medicines with you. These can be checked to see that you have the right medicines and that your inhaler technique is satisfactory.

Poor inhaler technique is a common reason for asthma medicines not working properly. If you are recording your peak flow readings, take them with you so that they can be discussed with your doctor or nurse.

During your check-up you might want to ask the following questions:

- Has my asthma attack resolved? (If not, you may need to be sent to hospital)

- Why did my asthma go out of control?

- Am I on the right asthma medicine?

- Do I use my inhaler correctly?

- What are the danger signs of uncontrolled asthma?

- Should I have an emergency supply of steroid tablets in case my asthma goes out of control? And how will I know when to take them?

- How can I make sure that I get emergency help next time this happens?

- Do I need to change my personal action (self-management) plan?

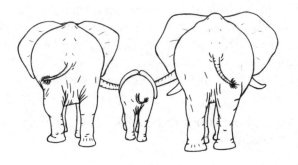

Glossary

Note. Terms that appear in *italic* in the definitions are also defined in this glossary.

acute   Short lasting. In medical terms this usually means lasting for hours or days, rather than for weeks or months.

adrenal glands   Important glands in the body, which produce a number of hormones to control the body systems. *Cortisol* and *cortisone* are two very important examples, and adrenaline is another.

airways   When we breathe in and out, air has to travel through hundreds of branching tubes, or airways, to and from the lung tissue (see Figure 1.1). In asthma the problem lies with these airways, which become narrow, preventing air from moving freely in and out of the lungs.

allergens   If you are 'allergic' to something, allergens are the tiny particles or substances to which you react when you come into contact with them.

allergic reaction   This is what happens when you come into contact with something to which you are allergic (an *allergen*). The allergic reaction varies from person to person and according to which part of your body reacts. For example, with grass pollen, an allergic reaction may take place in the lining of your nose (in which case you get *hay fever*), in the airways (causing asthma symptoms) or in the skin (causing *urticaria*, which is similar to nettle rash).

allergic rhinitis   An inflammation of the nasal airways. It occurs when an *allergen* such as dust or animal *dander* (particles of shed skin and hair) is inhaled by an individual *sensitised* to it. When caused by grass pollens, it is known as *hay fever*. It can be caused by tree pollens, moulds and *house dust mites*.

allergy   To have an allergy means to overreact to something in a harmful way when you come into contact with it. If you have an allergy to grass pollen you will have streaming eyes and nose, and sneezing if you come into contact with it (*hay fever*). Someone who is not allergic to grass pollen will not even notice grass pollen when they are in contact with it.

alveoli   These are the microscopic air spaces in the lungs which we refer to as the lung tissue. The airways get smaller and smaller as they divide into thousands of very tiny branches, and at the end of each of the smallest airways is an alveolus (plural = alveoli). Air mixes with the blood in the alveoli, and oxygen is taken in and carbon dioxide is passed out.

aminophylline   Generic name for one of the *reliever* type of drugs. Aminophylline can be taken by mouth or given by injection. There is no inhaled form. They are used less often nowadays.

anabolic steroids   Anabolic steroids are not used in the treatment of asthma. They cause the body to build up muscle, and because of this have been taken by some athletes to improve performance and strength. They should not be confused with *corticosteroids*, which are used to treat asthma and a number of other medical conditions.

anaphylaxis (anaphylactic attack)   A sudden, severe, potentially life-threatening *allergic reaction* caused, for example, by exposure to certain foods, insect stings or medicines. Symptoms include an itchy rash (hives), swelling (especially of the lips and face), difficulty breathing either because of swelling of the throat or a severe asthma attack, vomiting, diarrhoea, cramps and low blood pressure. An anaphylactic reaction should never be ignored and the emergency services should always be called.

antibodies   Substances produced by the body's immune system against 'attackers' such as infection.

anti-inflammatory drugs   Drugs that have an action against *inflammation*. Many diseases or conditions of the body – from asthma to arthritis to bowel disease – result in inflammation. Anti-inflammatory drugs reduce this inflammation and help the body to keep functioning as normal.

asthma register   This is a list kept of people with asthma, usually by a general practice. All practices have a list of patients registered with them. A proportion of those will have asthma, and they are listed in a separate register. This has advantages, the most important of which is that the practice can organise its care for those with asthma, keeping a check on treatments, and how often to review them.

atopic or atopy   To be 'atopic' is to have an allergic constitution. This means that in your make-up is the tendency to develop allergic, or atopic, conditions. The most important atopic conditions are *hay fever* and *eczema*. Asthma is strongly associated with atopy.

beta-agonists (also called beta-2-agonists, beta-stimulants or beta-2 stimulants). There are several names for this group of drugs, which can be very confusing! Short-acting beta-agonists bronchodilators (also called SABAs) are the most important group of *reliever* drugs, and they include Ventolin (salbutamol) and Bricanyl (terbutaline). Most often they are taken by inhaler, but they can also be given in tablet, liquid or injection form. Another group of inhaled beta-agonists – the long-acting beta-agonist bronchodilators (LABAs) – include the *longer-acting relievers* salmeterol (Serevent) and formoterol (Oxis and Foradil). These LABAs must not be used for asthma without also using inhaled *corticosteroid* inhalers. Therefore they are best used in combination formulations together with inhaled corticosteroids. (See also *bronchodilators* and *relievers*.)

bone age As children grow, their bones grow with them (of course!). As they grow, distinct changes can be traced in the bones by x-ray. If, for example, a child aged 7 years has an x-ray of the wrist, certain changes can be seen, corresponding to that age. In some children the bone age, as judged by x-rays, is ahead of or behind their actual age. This may be important in deciding whether a child's growth is being affected by a disease, or by certain medical treatments.

brand name All drugs in medicine have two names: their *generic name*, which is their true (chemical) drug name; and a brand name under which they are sold by their manufacturer. For example, Aspro, Anadin and Disprin are all brand names of the drug aspirin.

breath-activated inhaler (breath actuated) This is a type of inhaler device in which the drug is released only when a person breathes in. If no breath is taken, no drug is released from the device.

brittle asthma This is a severe variety of asthma and is not very common. Anyone with asthma might suffer an attack that comes on very quickly. However, people with brittle asthma can change, within minutes, from having no symptoms at all to having a very severe attack, despite taking regular treatment. Their attacks can prove very resistant to treatment. People with brittle asthma often need repeated hospital admissions, and very intensive treatment.

bronchi and **bronchioles** Bronchi are the main branches of the breathing tube (respiratory) system, taking air in and out of the lungs (see *airways*). Each time they branch, the diameter of the airway becomes smaller. The very smallest branches of the system are called bronchioles, and they end in air spaces called *alveoli*.

bronchial hyperreactivity   (also called bronchial hyperresponsiveness or BHR) This means an over-sensitivity in the airways, so that, when the *airways* come into contact with irritants (e.g. *allergens*, smoke, *viruses*) they overreact in a way that produces symptoms such as coughing and *wheezing*.

bronchiolitis   An important chest infection occurring in babies, usually in the winter months. It is caused by a *virus*, usually the respiratory syncytial virus (RSV), and often leaves the baby with coughing and *wheezing* for months or years afterwards.

bronchitis   This is a very common chest infection. The main symptom is cough, with the production of phlegm (sputum), usually yellow or green in colour. It may also cause *wheezing* and shortness of breath, and so can be confused with asthma. *Acute* bronchitis can occur in any age group at any time. *Chronic* bronchitis is a more serious condition of older people, usually smokers or those who have lived for years in polluted atmospheres.

bronchodilators   A medical term for *relievers*. They are called bronchodilators because they open up (dilate) the *airways* (*bronchi*). There are three main groups of bronchodilators, of which the *beta-agonists* (which include Ventolin [salbutamol] and Bricanyl [terbutaline]) are the most important.

candida infection   Another name for *thrush* (a fungal infection).

cardiac asthma   This book is about bronchial asthma. Cardiac asthma is a different condition resulting from heart failure. In heart failure, fluid becomes trapped in the lungs because the heart cannot pump strongly enough to clear it. The symptoms include shortness of breath and *wheezing*, as with bronchial asthma, but their cause (and treatment) is completely different. Cardiac asthma is not a term used very often these days, which is just as well, as it can be confusing.

chronic   In strictly medical terms, chronic means 'long lasting' or 'persistent'. In everyday use, many people using the word chronic mean severe or extreme. Both may apply. For example, chronic bronchitis by definition is persistent, but it often is severe.

chronic obstructive pulmonary disease (COPD)   This is a disease of the lungs that affects people over the age of 35 and is almost always due to smoking. Sometimes it is difficult to tell if someone has COPD or asthma. The medical history and *spirometry* may be helpful in diagnosing these people.

chronic severe asthma   another name for *brittle asthma*.

circadian rhythms The name for the body's natural rhythms during a period of 24 hours.

controllers Another name for *preventers*.

COPD see *chronic obstructive pulmonary disease.*

corticosteroids A particular group of chemicals that includes very important hormones, produced naturally by the body, and also many medicines used for a wide range of medical purposes. They are vital for the body's own action against infection and stress; in disease, when given as drugs, they are among the most effective agents available to doctors to treat inflammation. So, in asthma, which is a result of inflammation in the lining of the *airways*, they are the most effective treatment available. The name 'corticosteroid' is often shortened to 'steroid', causing people to confuse their asthma treatments with the *anabolic steroids* used for body building. Corticosterolids/steroids provide two of the most important treatments for asthma: the tablet form (prednisolone), which is mainly used in short courses and can be a life saver in acute attacks; and the inhaled form which, as AeroBec, Becotide, Becloforte, Filair, Flixotide, Pulmicort and Qvar, comprises the most important type of preventive treatment.

cortisol or cortisone A *corticosteroid* produced naturally by the body, in the *adrenal glands.*

cyanosis A blue discoloration of the skin, lips and tongue resulting from the blood carrying too little oxygen. In asthma attacks it is a sign of a very serious condition, and requires emergency treatment with oxygen.

dander (also called 'animal dander') Contents of animal hair, or fur, which cause an *allergic reaction.*

dehydration A condition in which the body is deficient in water. In asthma, this may occur over several hours, as a result of rapid breathing, vomiting, and difficulty in drinking usual amounts of fluid.

diurnal variation A change from one time of day to another 12 hours later, usually from early hours of the morning to evening. In this book we talk mainly about diurnal variation in peak flow readings, and this means the difference between readings taken first thing in the morning (which tend to be lower), and those taken in the evening (which tend to be higher).

dry-powder devices Inhalers in which the drug is delivered in the form of a powder, rather than an aerosol spray. The main types of dry-powder devices are the Diskus/Acuhaler (Figure 4.5), Aerolizer (Figure 4.6), Diskhaler (Figure 4.7), Easyhaler (Figure 4.8), Clickhaler (Figure 4.9),

Novolizer (Figure 4.10), Flexhaler (Figure 4.11), Pulvinal (Figure 4.12), Turbohaler (Figures 4.13 and Twisthaler (Figure 4.14).

early-onset asthma   Asthma that starts in childhood.

eczema   (also called *atopic* eczema) A red, itchy inflammation of the skin, sometimes with blisters and weeping. There are several different types. Atopic eczema is common in children and is associated with other *allergic* conditions, particularly *hay fever*, and asthma.

emphysema   An incurable lung disease in which the walls of the air sacs (*alveoli*) become damaged and enlarged. The lungs don't work very well and the person becomes increasingly short of breath. The main cause of emphysema is long-term regular smoking. This is a type of *chronic obstructive pulmonary disease*.

exercise-induced asthma   Symptoms of asthma brought on after several minutes of exercise, particularly running. Exercise is one of the most important triggers of asthma symptoms.

extrinsic asthma   An old term for asthma that is clearly triggered by some external factor, particularly *allergens* such as *house dust mite* and animal hair. The term '*atopic* asthma' is used in preference nowadays.

family history   The illnesses in other members of a family, including parents, grandparents, uncles, aunts and siblings.

general practitioner/GP   The family doctor.

gene   A unit of heredity, which helps to make up an individual's characteristics. Genes are contained on chromosomes in all the cells of the body. Each individual has his or her own set of millions of genes – half of which are inherited from the mother and half from the father.

generic name   The chemical, or true, name for a medicine. Different from the *brand name*, which is given by the company that produces it. Any one drug can have several brand names but only one generic name.

hay fever   A condition of the nose and eyes caused by *allergy* to grass pollen during the summer months. Sometimes the same allergy also results in asthma symptoms – so-called 'pollen' asthma. Hay fever is also known as 'seasonal *rhinitis*'.

house dust mite   A microscopic insect, correct name *Dermatophagoides pteronyssinus*. It survives by feeding on the dead scales of human skin. We all shed these in great numbers, continuously, and they collect in house dust, particularly in bedding. The house dust mite is the most important and common cause of *allergy*, *allergic rhinitis* and allergic asthma in the UK. Numbers are high all the year round, but especially so in the early winter months.

hygiene hypothesis A theory that people exposed to lots of different infective organisms are protected from developing *allergic* diseases; for example, people raised in a farming environment are exposed to a variety of organisms and suffer less from allergic disease.

hyperreactive See *bronchial hyperreactivity*.

hyperventilation (also known as over-breathing) This is breathing more often than the body needs for its oxygen requirements and for getting rid of carbon dioxide. It occurs most often in periods of tension, anxiety or over-excitement.

immune system The body's own defences against outside 'attackers', whether they are infections, injuries or other agents that are recognised as foreign (e.g. immunisations). The body's immune system reacts by attacking them, and producing *antibodies*, which give more long-lasting protection against future attackers of the same type. For example, in an attack of measles, the body's immune system fights off the infection after several days, but also produces antibodies that will protect for many years against a future attack.

inflammation The reaction of the body to some injury, infection or disease process. Generally, its purpose is to protect the body against the spread of injury or infection, but in some cases, as in asthma, the inflammation becomes *chronic*, and this tends to damage the body rather than protect it.

intrinsic asthma An old term for asthma that is not obviously triggered by any external agent, but tends to be continuous. The term 'non-*atopic* asthma' is used in preference nowadays.

late-onset asthma Asthma that begins in adult life, with no past history of its being a problem during childhood. Many people who seem to have late-onset asthma will give a *medical history* of being 'chesty' children, or having repeated 'bronchitis' or 'pneumonia' as children. This suggests that their asthma is recurring in adulthood, rather than appearing for the first time.

late reaction When people with asthma are exposed to triggers for their asthma, they may react within minutes with symptoms. This is usually easy to identify. However, there may be another 'late' reaction, which occurs approximately 6–10 hours afterwards. This is caused by a different set of reactions, but is every bit as important as the short-term reaction. Because of the time gap, it is more difficult to identify. It does not respond so well to *reliever* treatment as the short-term reaction.

leukotriene receptor antagonists (LTRAs)   LTRAs block one of the inflammatory pathways in the *airways* that cause asthma symptoms. They may be helpful in exercise-induced symptoms and *allergic rhinitis* if asthma is present. They are a tablet medicine, not an inhaler. They are used as additional treatment for asthma where people do not improve with steroid *preventers*.

litres per minute   (l/min) The reading on the peak flow meter is measured in litres per minute. It refers to the number of litres per minute that would be blown out of the lungs if someone could continue blowing at their peak flow rate.

long-acting relievers   There are two long-acting inhaled *bronchodilator* drugs: salmeterol (Serevent) and formoterol (Oxis or Aerolizer). They are used in addition to inhaled *corticosteroids/steroids* when asthma symptoms persist. They need be taken only twice daily.

lungs   The organs of breathing. The function of the lungs is to take oxygen into the bloodstream, and to get rid of the waste product, carbon dioxide, into the exhaled air.

medical history   Someone's past record of illnesses, symptoms and medical problems.

monilia infection   Another name for *thrush* or infection with candida.

morning dip   We all have a natural variation in our peak flow readings during day and night, which results in slightly lower readings in the morning than the evening. In asthma in general, and some people with asthma in particular, this pattern is very much exaggerated, so that a normal reading in the evening is followed by a pronounced 'dip' in the readings the following morning. This is recognised as an indication for changing treatment.

nasal polyp   See *polyp*.

NSAIDs   (full name: non-steroidal anti-inflammatory drugs) A class of drugs used extremely commonly for arthritis, other rheumatic conditions and generally for pain relief. Brufen, Nurofen, Froben, Ponstan, ibuprofen, indometacin, Feldene and Voltarol are well-known examples. All are related to aspirin, and in a few people can make asthma worse. They can also cause water retention, which may be a particular problem for people with heart or kidney disease.

occupational asthma   Asthma that results purely as a consequence of working in a particular environment.

oral steroids   *Corticosteroid* treatment given by mouth. Nearly always this is given as prednisolone tablets.

osteoporosis Thinning of the bones, which occurs as a result of overall loss of calcium from the body. The most important group affected by this is older women, who lose bone density more rapidly after their menopause. The results of osteoporosis are an increased risk of fractures, particularly of the spine and thigh bone.

over-breathing Another name for *hyperventilation*.

ozone A gas, related to oxygen, which is present in small amounts in the atmosphere.

passive smoking Breathing in smoke from another person's cigarette, cigar or pipe.

peak expiratory flow (PEF) In this book we also refer to peak flow rates, readings, charts, diaries, meters and monitoring! A PEF is a very simple but effective measure of how hard someone can blow air out of their lungs. The instrument used to measure it is a peak flow meter. If the *airways* are wide open, air can be blown out at a very high rate of *litres per minute*. If, as in asthma, the airways are narrowed, the PEF falls simply because air cannot be blown out at the same speed. A PEF reading is the measurement achieved on the scale of the meter; a peak flow chart is a record of PEF readings kept over a period of time, and a peak flow diary does the same, usually recording peak flow readings at particular times of day, and also keeping track of symptoms and treatment over the same time. Peak flow monitoring is usually carried out by the person with asthma. They have a home peak flow meter (available on National Health Service prescription) and can track their own condition, with assistance from their doctor or asthma nurse.

photochemical smog A very unhealthy atmosphere caused by a reaction between pollution near ground level and sunlight. This usually occurs in hot climates, where an urban environment is surrounded by mountains, which tend to trap the air (e.g. in places such as Los Angeles and Athens). It has occurred in the UK, especially in London. The smog contains gases that are damaging to the *lungs*, and can make asthma very much worse. These include *ozone*, particulate matter and oxides of nitrogen.

placebo A medicine that is inactive or ineffective. In clinical trials new drugs are tested against a placebo.

pleura Two layers of membrane surrounding and covering the lungs internally as a protection. Infection of the pleura results in pleurisy – a very painful condition.

polyp A small harmless growth, which arises from an internal lining of part of the body such as the lining of the bowel or the nose. Polyps in the nose are quite common in adults with asthma, particularly those whose asthma started later in life. (People with polyps may be *allergic* to aspirin.)

practice nurse   The term used for a nurse working in a general practice surgery, health centre or doctor's surgery.

preventers   (also known as controllers) Medicines that are taken to prevent the symptoms of asthma from occurring, rather than to relieve them when they do occur. The most important group of preventers is the inhaled *corticosteroid/steroid* drugs, described in Chapter 4.

propellants   These include CFCs (chlorofluorocarbons), which are now banned because of their effect on the environment, and HFAs (hydrofluoroalkanes), which have been developed to replace them.

puffer   A popular name for a metered-dose inhaler (MDI – Figure 4.1). The most commonly used inhalers release a puff of spray containing the drug when the canister is pressed.

relievers   A type of anti-asthma drug used intermittently for relieving symptoms and for emergency treatment. Relievers relax muscle spasm (tightness) around the *airways*, helping to open up the airways and relieve symptoms. Relievers are best used when needed rather than regularly. The most frequently prescribed reliever inhalers are Ventolin (salbutamol, albuterol) and Bricanyl (terbutaline). These are also known as short-acting beta-agonist (SABA) bronchodilators. Tablet forms of these two drugs are available, but their use is not recommended in asthma guidelines unless absolutely necessary.

remission   A period of time without symptoms or problems from a condition. In asthma the most likely time for a remission to occur is in late childhood. The condition may go into remission for many years, and treatment will not be required during this time. Asthma is such an unpredictable condition that it may go into remission at any time. However, the opposite also applies – after remission, it may return at any time.

rescue medicine   Another term for *reliever* medicine.

rhinitis   *Inflammation* of the lining of the nose – similar to the process of asthma in the *airways*. In the UK the most common reason for rhinitis is *allergy* to grass pollen (*hay fever* or seasonal rhinitis). The symptoms of rhinitis are runny nose, blocked nose, sneezing and itching.

rhinovirus   A type of virus known to cause the common cold and, in people with asthma, to provoke episodes of asthma with a cold (a 'cold going to the chest'), especially during the autumn and early winter months.

sensitise   A person becomes sensitised to an *allergen* when he or she produces *antibodies* to that *allergen*. *Allergy* tests that show the presence of these antibodies confirm that the person is sensitised, which is also called having an *atopic* status. When an atopic person gets symptoms after being exposed later to that allergen, he or she now has an allergy or is allergic to that allergen.

silent chest   When someone is having a severe asthma attack, they have difficulty breathing air in and out of the chest. Usually, during an asthma attack the person has very noisy, *wheezy* breathing that can be heard with a stethoscope. During a severe asthma attack, very little air is moving through the air passages. If the doctor or asthma nurse tries to listen to the breath sounds with a stethoscope during this severe attack, they may not hear anything – hence the name 'silent chest'.

skin-prick tests   Special tests to show whether a person has a tendency to *allergy*. Drops of solution containing *allergen* are placed on the forearm and the skin is pricked gently through the solution. A positive test occurs when a wheal, like a nettle rash, appears within 10 minutes. The tests are painless and inexpensive. The results of these tests may provide helpful information for the doctor or nurse.

spirometry   A test for lung function using an instrument called a spirometer. It is used to diagnose lung diseases such as asthma and *chronic obstructive pulmonary disease* (COPD).

steroids   see *corticosteroids*

tartrazine   An additive formerly found commonly in foods and soft drinks, but which is increasingly being omitted. It is probably the most important food additive implicated in asthma.

theophylline   Generic name for one of the *reliever* type of drugs. Theophylline can be taken by mouth or given by injection. There is no inhaled form. They are used less often nowadays.

thrush   (also called candida or monilia) A fungal infection of warm moist places in the body, particularly the mouth and skin folds. In asthma, thrush is an important side-effect of inhaled *corticosteroid* treatment. It is also a frequent consequence of a course of antibiotic treatment. Usually it is easily treatable.

topical (inhaled) steroids   Steroids that are inhaled or breathed in and so do not get absorbed directly into the bloodstream. This is an advantage, because it minimises the risk of side-effects. Inhaled topical steroids are used mainly in asthma (in inhaler devices) and in *allergic rhinitis* (e.g. *hay fever*).

trachea   The main windpipe, which begins at the level of the voice box (larynx), and goes into the top of the chest, where it divides into the *bronchi* (*airways*).

triggers   Factors that may bring on symptoms or attacks of asthma. They do not cause asthma.

twitchy airways   Another name for *bronchial hyperreactivity*.

uncontrolled asthma   The most important stage of asthma for you to recognise! This is when asthma begins to deteriorate, and heads towards an *acute* attack. If you can recognise it early, and take the right action, trouble will be prevented.

upper respiratory tract infection (URTI)   An infection of the ears, nose and throat. The best known example is the common cold. Almost all URTIs are caused by *viruses*. This means they take their own time to disappear, and they are rarely helped by giving antibiotics, which do not have any effect on virus infections.

urticaria   An allergic skin condition consisting of raised blotchy patches on the skin, looking very much like nettle rash

vasomotor rhinitis   *Rhinitis* triggered by cold weather; cold air causes a reaction in the lining of the nose.

virus   A microscopic organism, which multiplies in and attacks living cells, causing infections. There are many different groups of viruses and many thousands of different types of virus. The infections they cause vary enormously, from the trivial type to the fatal. Well-known examples are the common cold, influenza, measles, hepatitis and AIDS. Virus infections are important in asthma because they are the most common trigger of attacks. Colds going on to the chest, particularly in winter, are the triggers for many attacks. Virus infections are not helped by antibiotics.

wheeze/wheezing   The high-pitched or squeaky sound made when air is forced out of the *lungs* through narrowed *airways*.

work-aggravated asthma   Asthma that becomes worse at work because of the substances present there. (See also *occupational asthma*.)

Useful addresses, information and websites

The organisations given here are divided into sections – given in alphabetical order after the 'General' listing immediately below.

Please be aware that websites occasionally change their URLs. If you are unsuccessful using a URL given here, try searching for the organisation's name.

GENERAL

Admit
www.admit-inhalers.org

A website (only) with information for patients and healthcare professionals wanting information about asthma and COPD.

Allergy UK
Planwell House, LEFA Business Park, Edgington Way, Sidcup, Kent, DA14 5BH
Helpline: 01322 619 898
info@allergyuk.org
www.allergyuk.org

Dedicated to supporting people with allergy or intolerance conditions, and helping to educate health professionals who work with people with allergic conditions.

Anaphylaxis Campaign
1 Alexandra Road, Farnborough, Hants, GU14 6SX
Tel: 01252 546 100, Helpline: 01252 542 029
info@anaphylaxis.org.uk
www.anaphylaxis.org.uk

Campaigns for better awareness of life-threatening allergic reactions from food and drug allergies and to bee and wasp stings. Produces a wide range of educational newssheets and has an extensive support network.

Asthma and Allergy Foundation of America
www.aafa.org

A national network that works with volunteers, healthcare providers, government agencies and local communities to offer a variety of services, educational programmes and support.

Asthma Foundation Australia
www.asthmaaustralia.org.au

Provides advice, resources, education and training to support people with asthma, their carers, health professionals, first-aiders and the community.

Asthma UK
[England, Wales and Northern Ireland]
18 Mansell Street, London E1 8AA
Tel: 020 7786 4900
Helpline: 0300 222 5820
info@asthma.org.uk
www.asthma.org.uk

Produces excellent information and support for people with asthma and healthcare professionals, including:
- action plans for asthma management
- booklets and factfiles on any aspect of asthma
- frequently asked questions in a number of different languages
- a quarterly *Asthma Magazine* for members
- insurance (information and contact details if you are having problems obtaining travel insurance cover because of your asthma).

Also funds medical research.

Asthma UK Scotland
4 Queen Street, Edinburgh EH2 1JE
Tel: 0131 226 2544
Helpline: 0300 222 5820
scotland@asthma.org.uk
www.asthma.org.uk

Funds research and offers a range of information in different languages about coping with asthma. Helpline staffed by specialist asthma nurses. Has some support groups.

Asthma UK Wales
3rd floor, Eastgate House, 35–43 Newport Road, Cardiff CF24 0AB
Tel: 02920 435 400
Helpline: 0300 222 5820
wales@asthma.org.uk

Asthma UK Northern Ireland
Ground floor, Unit 2, College House, City Link Business Park,
Durham Street, Belfast BT12 4HQ
Tel: 0800 151 3035
Helpline: 0300 222 5820
ni@asthma.org.uk

Benefits Enquiry Line

This government agency and Helpline no longer exists. To find advice on
benefits for sick or disabled people go to the following site
www.gov.uk/benefit-adviser *and follow the relevant link(s)*

British Lung Foundation
73 75 Goswell Road, London EC1V 7ER
Tel: 020 7688 5555
Helpline: 03000 030 555
helpline@blf.uk.org
www.blf.org.uk

BLF has a network of support groups throughout the UK called Breathe Easy.
The website has all the contact details for these groups as well as a wide
range of information, which is also available in print. There is a quarterly
email newsletter called *Your BLF*.

British Thoracic Society (BTS)
17 Doughty Street, London WC1N 2PL
Tel: 020 7831 8778
bts@brit-thoracic.org.uk
www.brit-thoracic.org.uk

For UK asthma-management guidelines on air travel and diving, see
www.brit-thoracic.org.uk and follow the link to BTS Recommendations for
air travel, and to Guidelines for advice on diving.

Chest, Heart and Stroke organisations

Offer booklets, videos and DVDs on all aspects of chest, heart and stroke illness as well as community support groups. Some welfare grants available.

Scotland
3rd Floor, Rosebery House, 9 Haymarket Terrace, Edinburgh EH12 5EZ
Tel: 0131 225 6963
Advice line: 0845 077 6000
www.chss.org.uk

Northern Ireland
21 Dublin Road, Belfast BT2 7HB
Tel: 028 9032 0184
32 Ballinska Road
Springtown Industrial Estate
Derry / Londonderry
Tel: 028 7137 7222
www.nichs.org.uk

EFA (European Federation of Allergy and Airways Diseases Patients' Associations)
www.efanet.org

A network of organisations that cooperate with health professionals, scientists and other stakeholders to support people with allergies, asthma and COPD.

European Lung Foundation
442 Glossop Road, Sheffield S10 2PX
Tel: 0114 267 2875
info@europeanlung.org
www.europeanlung.org

Provides information to patients and health professionals on lung diseases, including asthma, COPD, cancer and tuberculosis.

European Patients Forum
Rue du Commerce 31, 1000 Brussels, BELGIUM
Tel: +32 2 280 2334
www.eu-patient.eu

An umbrella organisation that works with patient groups to ensure that people with life-long conditions have access to high-quality, patient-centred medical and social care.

GINA (Global Initiative for Asthma)
www.ginasthma.org

Works with healthcare and public health professionals to reduce the prevalence, morbidity and mortality of asthma.

Mark Levy's website
www.consultmarklevy.com

Midlands Asthma and Allergy Research Association (MAARA)
PO Box 1057, Leicester LE2 3GZ
Tel: 0116 247 9888
enquiries@maara.org
www.maara.org

A research and support association offering advice and information for people with asthma and allergies, their families as well as health professionals.

National Health Service
The Department of Health website is available via: www.gov.uk
https://www.gov.uk/government/organisations/department-of-health

Prescription Pricing Authority
Tel: 0300 330 1341
www.nhsbsa.nhs.uk/

Manages the Prescription Prepayment Scheme: by prepaying for a 'season ticket' – a Prescription Prepayment Certificate – covering 3 months or a year, money can be saved on prescribed medicines if you need more than 3 medicines in 3 months or more than 13 medicines in a year.

Scottish Intercollegiate Guidelines Network (SIGN)
Healthcare Improvement Scotland
Gyle Square, 1 South Gyle Crescent, Edinburgh EH12 9EB
Tel: 0131 623 4720
www.sign.ac.uk

Produces guidelines across many medical specialities, including several on asthma: 6, 33, 38, 63 and 101.

Royal National Institute for the Blind
www.rnib.org.uk
Helpline: 0303 123 9999

Sells different coloured raised labels called 'Bumpons', which you can attach to inhalers to help identify them more easily.

UK Inhaler Group
www.respiratoryfutures.org.uk/programmes/uk-inhaler-group

Website giving useful information about the use of inhaled medications.

ALERTING SYSTEM

MedicAlert
The MedicAlert Foundation, 327 Upper Fourth Street,
Milton Keynes MK9 1EH
Tel: 01908 951045
info@medicalert.org.uk
www.medicalert.org.uk

A global charity that provides emergency identification with body-worn jewellery for people with hidden medical conditions and allergies. There is a 24-hour emergency telephone which accepts reverse-charge calls; can access personal details from anywhere in the world.

CHILDREN AND SCHOOLS

Department of Education

The publication *Supporting Pupils at School with Medical Conditions* (updated 2014) (reference: 1448-2005DCL-EN) can be downloaded from National Archives on the government website: https://www.gov.uk/government/consultations/supporting-pupils-at-school-with-medical-conditions

ECZEMA

National Eczema Society
11 Murray Street, London NW1 9RE
Tel: 020 7281 3553
Helpline: 0800 089 1122 Mon–Fri 8am–8pm
www.eczema.org

A charitable organisation specifically for people with eczema; provides practical help, information and support.

EDUCATION

Boots the Chemist
www.ebc-indevelopment.co.uk/asthma/index.html

Contains information on the lungs and asthma, linked to the national educational curriculum.

INTERNET SEARCH ENGINES

These are just a few of the more commonly used sites in the UK:
Ask Jeeves: www.ask.com
Chrome: www.googlechrome
Google: www.Google.com
Yahoo: www.yahoo.com

MANUFACTURERS OF ASTHMA MEDICINES AND EQUIPMENT

AstraZeneca (UK) Ltd
Tel: 0800 783 0033
www.astrazeneca.co.uk
- Accolate tablets
- Flexhaler
- Turbohaler

Boehringer Ingelheim Ltd
Ellesfield Avenue, Bracknell, Berkshire RG12 8YS
medinfo@bra.boehringer-ingelheim.co.
www.boehringer-ingelheim.co.uk
- Metered-dose inhaler
- Respimat

Canday Medical Limited
PO Box 962, Newmarket CB8 1AE
www.2tonetrainer.net
- 2tonetrainer

Chiesi Pharmaceuticals
333 Styal Road, Manchester, M22 5LG
Tel: 0161 488 5555
info@chiesi.uk.com
www.chiesi.uk.com
- Pulvinal
- Fostair

Clement Clarke International Ltd
Edinburgh Way, Harlow, Essex CM20 2TT
Tel: 01279 414 969
resp@clement-clarke.com
www.clement-clarke.com

Suppliers of peak flow meters, spacers, Trainhaler, In-Check Dial and nebulisers.

Epipen
www.epipen.co.uk

Gives useful information about Epipen autoinjectors.

Fyne Dynamics Ltd.
1 Horsecroft Place, Pinnacles, Harlow CM19 5BT
Tel: 01279 423 423
www.fyne-dynamics.com
- Mag-Flo Inhaler Trainer
- Pinnacle Peak Flow Meter

GlaxoSmithKline
980 Great West Road, Brentford, Middlesex TW8 GS
www.gsk.com
- Accuhaler
- Aerochamber spacer devices (sole distributor in UK)
- Babyhaler
- Metered-dose inhaler
- Volumatic

Merck Sharp & Dohme Ltd. (MSD)
Hertford Road, Hoddesdon EN11 9BU
Tel: 01992 467 272
www.msd-uk.com
- Montelukast tablets

MIMS
Bridge House, 69 London Road, Twickenham TW1 3SP
www.mims.co.uk

Mundi Pharma International Ltd
Unit 194, Cambridge Science Park, Milton Road, Cambridge CV4 0AB
Tel: 01223 424 211
www.mundipharma.com
- Flutiform

Napp Pharmaceuticals Group
Cambridge Science Park, Milton Road, Cambridge CV4 0AB
Tel: 01223 424 444
napp.co.uk
- Flutiform

nSpire Health
8 Harforde Court, John Tate Road, Hertford SG13 7NW
Tel: 01992 526 300
info@nspirehealth.com
www.nspirehealth.com
- Nspire Peak Flow Meter
- Pocket Chamber
- Piko (electronic peak flow meter)

Sanofi UK
One Onslow Street, Guildford GU1 4YS
Tel: 01483 505 515
www.sanofi.co.uk
- Tilade cfc free inhaler
- Intal cfc

Takeda UK Ltd
Building 3, Glory Park, Glory Park Avenue, Wooburn Green
High Wycombe, Bucks HP10 0DF
Tel: 01628 537 900
www.takeda.co.uk
- Metered-dose inhaler

Teva UK Ltd
Ridings Point, Whistler Drive, Castleford WF10 5HX
Tel: 01977 628 500
www.tevauk.com
- Autohaler
- Easi-breathe
- Metered-dose inhaler
- DuoResp Spiromax

Trudell Medical International
Biocity Nottingham, Pennyfoot Street, Nottingham NG1 1GF
Tel: 0115 912 4380
www.trudellmedical.com
- AeroChamber manufacturer

Williams Medical Supplies
Craiglas House, Maerdy Industrial Estate, Rhymny NP22 5PY
Tel: 01685 844 7393 500
Website: www.wms.co.uk
- MicroPeak Peak Flow Meter

MEDICINES INFORMATION

British National Formulary
www.bnf.org

Electronic Medicines Compendium (eMC)
www.medicines.org.uk/emc

For information on medicines available in the UK.

OCCUPATIONAL ASTHMA

British Occupational Health Research Foundation (BOHRF)
www.bohrf.org.uk

A non-profit, grant-making charity that closed down in 2013 but whose website provides access to research reports on occupational health.

ORGANISATIONS FOR PROFESSIONALS

Education for Health
The Athenaeum, 10 Church Street, Warwick CV34 4AB
Tel: 01926 493 313
www.educationforhealth.org

An educational charity which provides training for health professionals in the care of their patients with cardiovascular, respiratory and allergic disease in general practice and the hospital setting. The courses are internationally recognised.

GINA (Global Initiative for Asthma)
www.ginasthma.org

Works with healthcare professionals and public health officials worldwide to reduce the prevalence of asthma and its impact on those with the condition.

Health and Safety Executive HQ

Redgrave Court, Merton Road, Bootle, Merseyside L20 7HS

www.hse.gov.uk

Offers information and advice about health and safety regulations in the workplace for people with asthma, employers and health professionals.

National Institute for Health and Care Excellence (NICE)

10 Spring Gardens, London SW1A 2BU

Tel: 0300 323 0140

www.nice.org.uk

Provides national guidance on the promotion of good health and the prevention and treatment of ill health. Patient information leaflets are available for each piece of guidance issued.

Primary Care Respiratory Society UK

Unit 2, Warwick House, Kingsbury Road, Curdworth

Sutton Coldfield B76 9EE

Tel: 01675 477600

www.pcrs-uk.org

An independent charity representing primary care health professionals. Publishes the *Primary Care Respiratory Journal* (www.thepcrj.org)

POLLEN

The National Pollen and Aerobiology Research Unit

Charles Darwin Building, University of Worcester, Henwick Grove

Worcester WR2 6AJ

Tel: 01905 855 411

www.pollenuk.co.uk

Provides information about pollen counts and pollen monitoring, useful for people with hay fever.

Metereological Office

FitzRoy Road, Exeter EX1 3PB

Tel: 0370 900 0100 or 01392 885 680

Provides pollen forecasts for up to five days ahead.

SMOKING AND STOPPING SMOKING

ASH (Action on Smoking and Health)

6th Floor, Suites 59–63, New House, 67–68 Hatton Garden
London EC1N 8JY
Tel: 020 7404 0242
www.ash.org.uk

A campaigning charity working to eliminate the harm caused by tobacco.

Quitnow (Smokefree NHS)

https://quitnow.smokefree.nhs.uk

Offers advice on giving up smoking, including to schools. Can put people in touch with local support groups. Has free same-day advice on email.

SPORTS AND DRUGS

UK Anti-Doping

Fleetbank House, 2–6 Salisbury Square, London EC4Y 8AE
Tel: 020 7842 3450
www.ukad.org.uk

A useful drug information database of permitted or prohibited drugs for a wide range of sports.

World Anti-Doping Agency

www.wada-ama.org

Has very strict regulations on which drugs may be used in competitive sport.

Flying and Scuba diving

Information available on national recommendations at British Thoracic Society website: www.brit-thoracic.org.uk

Full address is under the 'General' heading in this section.

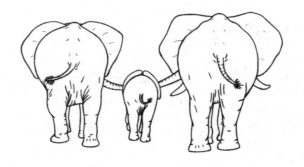

Index

Entries in **bold** indicate a diagram or illustration; entries with an italic *g* at the end indicate a glossary definition.

*Have you found this book useful and practical?
If so, you may be interested in other titles from our
award-winning 'Answers at your fingertips' series.*

Answers at your fingertips

'Woe betide any clinicians or nurses whose patients have read this invaluable source of down-to-earth information when they have not.' – *The Lancet*

Our best selling series, *Answers at your fingertips*, seeks to help those who, having been diagnosed with a condition, have countless questions that need answering. These essential handbooks answer all the questions that patients want to know about their health and condition.
The formula for the series follows a question-and-answer format, with real questions from sufferers and their families answered by medical experts at the top of their fields, without the jargon of medical texts.
All these books are packed full of practical information for patients and their families. Topics covered range from diagnosis to treatment, and from relationships to welfare entitlements.

'Contains the answers the doctor wishes he had given if only he'd had the time.' – Dr Thomas Stuttaford, *The Times*

Titles currently available:
*Acne • Allergies • Asthma • Breast Cancer •
COPD • Alzheimer's & other dementias • Type 1 Diabetes •
Type 2 Diabetes • Epilepsy• Epilepsy and your child •
Eczema • Gout • Heart Health • High Blood Pressure • IBS •
Kidney Dialysis & Transplants • Migraine & other headaches •
Motor Neurone Disease • Menopause • Multiple Sclerosis • Osteoporosis •
Parkinson's • Psoriasis • Sexual Health for Men • Stroke •*

For current availability of the *Answers at your fingertips* range,
please contact us on 01278 427800 or:
**Class Publishing, The Exchange, Express Park,
Bridgwater, TA6 4RR**

The *Class Health* Feedback Form

We hope that you found this *Class Health* book helpful. We always appreciate readers' opinions and would be grateful if you could take a few minutes to complete this form for us.

1. **How did you acquire your copy of this book?**
    - ☐ From my local library
    - ☐ Read an article in a newspaper/magazine
    - ☐ Found it by chance
    - ☐ Recommended by a friend
    - ☐ Recommended by a patient organisation/charity
    - ☐ Recommended by a doctor/nurse/advisor
    - ☐ Saw an advertisement

2. **How much of the book have you read?**
    - ☐ All of it
    - ☐ More than half of it
    - ☐ Less than half of it

3. **Which copies/chapters have been most helpful?**

4. **Overall, how useful to you was this *Class Health* book?**
    - ☐ Extremely useful
    - ☐ Very useful
    - ☐ Useful

5. **What did you find most helpful?**

6. **What did you find least helpful?**

....

....

....

7. **Have you read any other health books?**

☐ Yes

☐ No

If yes, which subjects did they cover?

....

....

....

How did this *Class Health* book compare?

☐ Much better

☐ Better

☐ About the same

☐ Not as good

8. **Would you recommend this book to a friend?**

☐ Yes

☐ No

Thank you for your help. Please send your completed form to:

FREEPOST
Class Learning

(No postcode required. No stamp needed if posted in the UK)

Title Prof/Dr/Mr/Mrs/Ms ....

Surname.. First name................................

Address ....

Town.. Postcode ....

Country...

☐ Please add my name and address to receive details of related books.
   (Please note, we will not pass on your details to any other company).